In the Shadow of Medicine:
Remaking the Division of Labor in Health Care

Arnold Birenbaum

St. John's University

GENERAL HALL, INC.
Publishers
5 Talon Way
Dix Hills, New York 11746

In the Shadow of Medicine:
Remaking the Division of Labor in Health Care

GENERAL HALL, INC.
5 Talon Way
Dix Hills, New York 11746

Publisher: Ravi Mehra
Consulting Editor: Anand Sinha
Composition: *Graphics Division,* General Hall, Inc.

LIBRARY OF CONGRESS CATALOG CARD NUMBER: **90–80203**

ISBN: 0-930390-27-X [paper]
0-930390-28-8 [cloth]

Manufactured in the United States of America

Dedicated to the One I Love

Contents

Introduction　　　　　　　　　　**1**

The Sociology of Occupations and Professions 5, The Social
Context 11, References 15

**1　Professions and Professionals
　　in Modern Times**　　**16**

The Idea of Sovereign Professions 25, The Professionalization
of Medicine in a Historic Context 26, The Contemporary Context for Paramedical Professions 29, References 31

**2　The Growth of Bureaucratic
　　Medicine**　　**32**

New Practitioners, New Relationships 33, New Demands and
Health Care Planning 36, Cost Containment and Task Shifting
42, The Crisis in Pharmacy 43, Origins of the Crisis 47, The
Decline of the Community Pharmacy 48, Automation 49,
Physician Extenders 50, New Patterns of Recruitment 51,
Communication among Pharmacists 51, Social Mobility
Within Bureaucratized Health Care 52, References 53

**3　Reinventing Primary Care:
　　The Training of Physician
　　Extenders**　　**56**

Education and Training 59, The Making of a Professional
Identity 62, Independent Judgment 65, Evaluation of Perfor-
mance 68, Second Thoughts: the AMA Reviews Control 71,
References 73

4 Social Approval of Physician Extenders and Institutional Barriers 76

Physician Approval 79, Relationships between Physician Extenders and Physicians 79, New Forms of Utilization 82, Creating Credibility 84, Patient Satisfaction and the Management of Impressions 90, Some Anticipated and Unanticipated Problems 94, Role Expansion and Legal Problems 96, Concerning Direct Payment 97, References 99

5 Efforts to Change the Image of Pharmacy 102

Pharmacy against Itself 103, The War of Words in Pharmacy 105, Image Changing Activities 105, Identification of a New Direction 105, Delegation of Routine Tasks 106, The Need for Continuing Education 107, Avoiding False Opportunities and Seeking In-Depth Knowledge 108, Raising the Public Image of the Profession 111, Increasing Professionalism in the Associations 113, Professionalism and Reprofessionalization 114, References 116

6 Cultural Authority and Boundary-Work: Creating Markets for Clinical Pharmacy 118

Expanding the Boundaries of Pharmacy 121, Creating Awareness of a Service 121, Eliminating Restrictions on Practice 123, Upgrading of Responsibilities 124, Remuneration for Upgraded Activities 125, Aggressive Marketing of Services 127, Innovative Projects 128, The Dialectics of Professional Development 133, References 135

7 The Expansion of Pharmacy and the Shortfall in Clinical Positions: Discontinuities Between Production and Distribution 140

Reforms in Education and Opportunities to Practice Clinical Pharmacy 143, Reinventing Pharmacy Education and Educators 146, Physician Response 148, The Material Foundation of the Physician's Authority 149, References 154

8 Current Behavior and Future Directions 156

Future Directions 156, Physician Assistants 156, Nurse Practitioners 157, Clinical Pharmacy 160, The New Division of Labor 163, References 166

Name Index 167

Subject Index 172

List of Tables

Table 4.1   Equivalence in Quality of Care
Provided by Nurse Practitioners (NPs)
and Physicians (MDs), 1971–1986   86

Table 4.2   Difference in Quality of Care Provided
by Nurse Practitioners (NP) and
Physicians (MD), 1974–1982   87

INTRODUCTION

Max Weber, in writing about the relationship between faith and courage in the *Protestant Ethic and the Spirit of Capitalism*, demonstrated that, under certain conditions, human groups with members not noted for military skill or tradition could act bravely. Armed with a strong consciousness of mission and strong in-group support, the founders of ascetic Protestantism were willing to take risks. In order to receive a sign that they were among the saved, they often broke with traditional practices and were successful, thereby reassuring themselves that they would have a place in the next world. By virtue of their success, these religious rebels helped to remake the world along modern lines. And, of course, they changed their position in society as well.

In far less dramatic ways, challenged by changing social and economic arrangements, members of professions and occupations today are placed in a similar position to the Protestant Divines of the seventeenth century. Active elements seek to reverse or alter trends that create a problematic or limited future for their profession. Inspired by an alternative vision, they may seize the opportunity to lift up the entire profession by its bootstraps.

When members of an occupation engage in a collective mobility project, anomalous events occur. In some instances the leadership, for greater autonomy as well as responsibility, may break with their sponsors. In other cases, activists may find resistance from within and outside the profession.

In the late 1960s, with the social responsibility for health care in America clearly and securely in the hands of the medical profession, an elite group within the profession sought to correct for the overdevelopment of specialization in the field. New roles were created to extend the care provided by physicians; this delegation of responsibilities, in the main, occurred in

1

primary care, the least remunerative and least prestigious branch of medicine. Physician extenders or physician associates, as they were designated, were at first happy with their new roles. Once content to be within the shadow of medicine, by the 1980s, the nurse practitioners, most of them women and former nurses, now also sought a place for themselves in the sun. They sought a future with greater independence in their practice of health care, based on a partnership with medicine rather than a subordinate role.

Pharmacy is another profession in which activists are attempting to ensure a better future. Facing a crisis of purpose, some in the field have attempted to expand the role of the pharmacist in a clinical direction, suggesting that physicians and nurses learn to regard pharmacists as experts on the effects and effectiveness of drugs. In addition, the clinically oriented see a future in which pharmacists will delegate their typical dispensing functions to technicians and in so doing become free to educate and instruct patients on how to administer medications, thus increasing patient compliance with prescriptions. Clinical work for the pharmacist would be consultive in nature.

> In the ideal system, patient education would be a standard service of pharmacists that would go with dispensing every prescription. National organizations representing medicine and pharmacy would jointly develop educational protocols, according to therapeutic category, for the pharmacist to follow unless the physician directed otherwise. . . . Coupled with appropriate information from the physician (including diagnosis), the protocols would allow the pharmacist to exercise professional judgment in each instructional encounter. The pharmacist could make sure that the patient comprehends key information, thereby enhancing the patient's responsibility for his treatment. For certain patients (like the first-time insulin user), the physician could prescribe special in-depth instruction which the pharmacist would provide to the patients for a fee. (Zellmer 1976, 535)

In seeking to shape the future of pharmacy, adherents of the clinical movement predict that by the year 2000, pharmacy will be a personal health-care service. They envision pharmacists collaborating with physicians and nurses, as well as having a direct professional relationship with patients and their families (Lamy 1975). Moreover, at the level of national association meetings, the profession of medicine and the profession of pharmacy will convene as peers, collectively developing protocols to enhance patient compliance.

Pharmacy will have not only greater cultural authority under this ideal system but also a new form of social organization and division of labor. Pharmacists will become applied clinical pharmacologists, assisting a medical specialty that is in short supply. Colleges of pharmacy will be reorganized to reflect this new responsibility, training both clinical pharmacists with the first practice degree a doctorate (Pharm. D.), and technicians to attend to the distributive functions of pharmacy (Francke 1975; Schwartz 1975).

Despite these dreams of new responsibilities and authority, sociologists and other students of occupations and professions have shown little interest in the clinical movement in pharmacy. Until now, sociologists have conceived of pharmacy as a marginal profession, mixing business and professional values (Denzin 1972), and have regarded this combination as more or less constant, not subject to change. Moreover, since the organization and policies of pharmaceutical corporations have strongly affected the practice of pharmacy in the United States, the independence of pharmacy has often been questioned, just as the professional autonomy of engineering has been questioned because of its extreme dependence on the captains of industry. These built-in contradictions only make the study of this new movement in pharmacy all the more intriguing and important, since the replacement of craft production by bureaucratic and capital-intensive forms of organization is a major theme in labor history and the sociology of work.

Under these social conditions, how has a movement toward remaking the profession of pharmacy into a clinical practice emerged? Is it possible for a licensed but subordinate profession, with diverse practices in communities, hospitals, and nursing homes, to remake itself? Will a qualitatively different breed of pharmacist, a specialist with new responsibilities, appear in the field? Will applied clinical pharmacology extract itself from pharmacy and enter the domain of medicine? Or, as the advocates of clinical pharmacy have it, will the entire profession simply be upgraded educationally in order to keep pace with the knowledge, advancements in medicine, and greater sophistication and responsibility found in nursing?

The story of the rise of clinical pharmacy is not just interesting simply because it is heroic — here is a craft resisting the possibility of becoming obsolete — but also because it has a pretentious quality to it. Some of the steps advocated by adherents of clinical pharmacy appear to be no more than transparent efforts to increase the status of the profession and the income of its members.

The growth of the hospital and increasing medical specialization as major organizational forms for delivery of health care accounts for the search for new ways to cut costs while ensuring quality care. Planners became increasingly concerned in the 1970s with ways to reduce hospital admissions and decrease the length of stay. They also suggested that physicians did not have to evaluate and treat minor illnesses, educate and screen patients in order to prevent serious illness (e.g., hypertension), and monitor long-term posthospitalization recovery.

The times seem right for the development of new practices and new practitioners in the health-care field. Under the sponsorship of medicine, two middle-level health care practitioner roles — physician assistant and nurse practitioner — have been created. The new roles have followed the long-established trend of doctors to delegate tasks to nurses. From the point of view of the physician, the extenders represent either a potential competitor or a new way to expand one's practice. State laws on medical practice and nursing have been amended to provide for the delegation of tasks to these physician extenders as long as they function under a physician's supervision and control.

A new division of labor is emerging in which physicians may have to share responsibility for health-care with the new practitioners rather than simply delegating tasks. Given the increasing sense of responsibility found among nurse practitioners and physician assistants, and the need to exercise independent judgment, a call for a shift in decision-making power to the health care team is likely to emerge. To what extent these new health-care practitioners have the opportunity to shape decision making and gain control over their work situation is a major research question in the field of medical sociology.

The capacity of the new practitioners to exercise independent judgment is not only a result of their training and the environments in which they work, but an outcome of the way in which their roles are defined. When they are permitted to carry their own caseload and follow patients on a long-term basis, they become experts on their patients. Yet patients may impute limited skills to nurse practitioners or physician assistants by virtue of their position in the hospital's organizational hierarchy. To what extent does their skill and dedication (i.e., professionalism) override their location in the division of labor and lack of opportunity to shape it?

The remaking of the division of labor in health care is also a process that provides the sociologist with an opportunity to examine critically some of the major models developed on the origins of professions in advanced industrial societies. From this excellent research site it is possible to locate the structural conditions that account for the emergence of an occupation into an autonomous profession. And it is possible to learn more about how traditional occupations become threatened, are able to reform, and then develop new markets for the modern version of their traditional practices. Thus a study of changes in health-care delivery contributes to the generic understanding of how people live and work in society.

The Sociology of Occupations and Professions

The study of occupations and professions has a long and distinguished tradition in sociology. In the nineteenth century, the founders of the discipline — Marx, Weber, and Durkheim — were sensitive to the complex ways in which industrialization, economic development, and modern attitudes were changing relationships between occupational groups, between providers and consumers, and between employers and employees. As early as 1848, Marx observed that "the bourgeoisie has stripped of its halo every occupation hitherto honoured and looked up to with reverent awe." According to Marx and other social analysts of his day, the reduction of independence entailed when a person worked for wages (instead of selling a product or receiving a fee for a service) engendered a sense of loss in prestige and power. In turn, the manager and organizer of the labor of others developed a strong sense of mastery; and, as Alexis deTocqueville observed during his travels in America, the development of industry based on mass distribution created a new aristocracy that seemed born to command:

> While the workman concentrates his faculties more and more upon the study of a single detail, the master surveys an extensive whole, and the mind of the latter is enlarged in proportion as that of the former is narrowed. In a short time the one will require nothing but physical strength without intelligence; the other stands in need of science, and almost of genius to ensure success. This man resembles more and more the administrator of a vast empire; that man a brute. (Tocqueville 1945, 1:169)

Content with pointing out the unintended consequences of democracy, Tocqueville mistook the appearance of narrowness and docility for the complete person. In the nineteenth century, workers often remained convinced that they too could manage and organize industry—sometimes they organized to that end, sometimes they studied together to improve their minds and become masters of their world. Much of this activity took place away from the workplace and could be hidden from the eyes of even such a formidable observer as Tocqueville.

The sociologist today faces unexpected barriers when attempting to get a close look at work and working. Professions, in particular, develop internal arrangements for dealing with the outside world, including the social sciences, that limit access. To study a profession undergoing change requires contact with practitioners in the field, an opportunity that cannot be taken for granted. The presence of external threats or a sharp decline in the fortunes of a profession should provide an opportunity for social science research. Yet those points in history, the professions, recognizing their crisis, become introspective and create blue-ribbon panels of thoughtful and learned outsiders to describe and evaluate conditions in the field. The Flexner Report in medicine and the Millis Report in pharmacy represent the products of two self-sustained study commissions. While not all physicians or pharmacists welcomed or benefited from these panels, there was "inside" sponsorship from at least some segments of these professions.

Without such sponsorship, a number of barriers face the social scientist interested in professions in flux. The first personal and professional problem for the "uninvited" sociologist emerges when he or she considers doing a case study. Practitioners of any occupation often convey amazement and surprise that anyone outside the profession could be interested in their problems and aspirations. Moreover, since professions have associations to represent them, they develop home-grown equivalents to social analysts who assess where the field is going at a particular point in time. Aside from these full-time internal experts on the profession, each member of the field feels more knowledgeable than any outsider about trends and issues. Specializing in the study of the family, or even ethnic group conflict, does not produce the same structure of expertise as attempts at a firsthand study of professions and occupations.

A second problem emerges in the study of work groups of any kind and relates to the highly developed social cohesion found in these communities. When work groups form tightly bound communities, contact with an outsider may be used to reinforce these loyalties. The tension between observer and observed is especially evident in the way in which the work of the social scientist can be subject to ridicule. In doing field research of any kind, sociologists are often the butt of inside jokes or are otherwise tested by community or group members. In work groups, these activities take the form of initiating the newcomer, revealing a great deal about the social solidarity of the membership. These on-the-job activities do not indicate how tacit knowledge is used by the community at work, only how it is transmitted from cohort to cohort.

A third problem emerges when studying consulting professions with their specific terminology and skills available only to those who study and train in professional schools. Sociologists face a moderate amount of uncertainty because they have not been through the schooling of the practitioner, where knowledge, ability, and motivation peculiar to the profession is acquired. By definition, the professional takes care of other people's problems, using a base of knowledge foreign to the layperson. Therefore, it is reasonable to ask, How can one describe and explain what is not fully understood? The technical side of the profession remains a mystery to most outsider observers; the social side of professional behavior, however, is not that esoteric. Many of the activities and attitudes of members of the profession represent attempts to receive a favorable opinion from others. Being an expert is a social construction as much as it is a ratification of the demonstration of technical effectiveness. Occupations, somewhat like individuals, strive for recognition and the opportunity to get others dependent on them for services. They may invoke claims of superiority even when the proficiency of the performers has little potential to improve or when objective measures of productivity show little change in output. Professions often compete with one another for the legal right to provide a valued service. Under these conditions, the social side of professions is laid bare; and here sociologists are, perhaps, on most firm grounds, helping to sharpen our understanding of society and occupations.

Building on various orientations, sociologists have been able to show how each profession seeks legitimation, or a kind of popular *and* official recognition of its stature in society. Organized skepticism, an intellectual trait shared by sociologists and journalists who do investigative work, encourages this kind of inquiry. Sociology and investigative journalism do part company on the issue of whether scholarly analysis and presentation and theoretical contributions are necessary. Paul Starr provides a clear illustration of this orientation and what must be attended to when examining a profession from a sociological perspective.

> Professional claims, of course, should not be taken simply on face value. The rewards of professional status encourage would-be and even established professions to invent or elaborate credentials, sciences, and codes of ethics in bids for recognition.

Rather than as indicators of professional status, such features should be seen as the means of legitimating professional authority, achieving solidarity among practitioners and gaining a grant of monopoly from the state. Occupations may or may not succeed, depending on their means of collective organization and the receptivity of the public and the government. In this sense, professionalism represents a form of occupational control rather than a quality that inheres in some kind of work. But professionalism is also a kind of solidarity, a source of meaning in work, and a system of regulating belief in modern societies. (Starr 1982, 16)

A fourth problem confronts the investigator who seeks to study the structure and process of professionalization or reprofessionalization because of the groundwork laid by other sociologists. The model for how an occupation gains responsibility and autonomy is almost exclusively derived from the history and sociology of the rise of medicine as a sovereign profession. A dominant profession without peer in the United States, although not quite so sovereign in other countries, medicine has been observed and analyzed frequently from a sociological perspective. Moreover, despite the much-noted observation that medicine in other countries has been organized on terms very different from those found in the United States, the idea of connecting professionalization with private practice is so strong that when other professions are analyzed, they are seen as inferior unless the practitioners are self-employed. Since American medicine reached its ascendant position under specific historical conditions, and has set the pattern of development for other occupations, its rise provides some striking analogies with events in other professions.

Medicine, in turn, is a reality that all other professions, particularly those in the health-care field, must reckon with. So dominating is medicine in the field that the study of the secondary health professions must appear to be based on contentment with or a desire to consort with the mediocre. To consider nursing and pharmacy as professions in the same way as one considers law and medicine professions seems to be almost an error in judgment. Yet even while the yearnings and struggles currently seen in nursing and pharmacy were initiated by medicine, it can be argued that these quests for greater responsibility and autonomy would have come about even if medicine did not exist.

And this brings us to the fifth problem in undertaking an investigation of how a profession attempts to leave its origins or remake itself to ensure a better future. While the power of physicians to call the shots in health care is not as great as it once was, they have successfully resisted being dominated, as other artisans and craftsmen were, by the corporation or the state (Starr 1982, 25). As the leading experts on health care matters, large or small, physicians are both the model for professional autonomy to be emulated by other health care providers and the residing powers who must be convinced of the merit of reassigning tasks and authority if the other occupations are to acquire the same or similar degrees of control over their work in the health-care field. As a powerful profession, American medicine is in a similar position to England in the nineteenth century as the first industrialized country in relation to the rest of the world. Sought after strenuously by many countries, industrialization could be impeded or accelerated by the nation in which it first successfully appeared in the world. British industrialization shaped the economies of nonindustrialized countries, by ruining a region or a nation's traditional means of production, turning it into a market for cheap consumer goods or using it as a source of materials extracted from the ground or grown.

The profession of medicine is in a hegemonic position in the health-care field, so much so that the other professions are not masters of their fate. The profession of medicine has shaped the paramedical professions as it wishes, calling into being broad nonclinical specialists of various kinds (e.g., pathology, radiology, anesthesiology) or those who perform narrowly defined and purely technical roles (e.g., blood technician, physical therapist); it can relegate unwanted but necessary tasks to other professions (e.g., the formulation and dispensing of medicines) and deny others the right to give advice or interpret procedures and diseases, even when the provider of the service is in direct and frequent contact with the patient.

Despite all these obstacles to investigation, some penetrating concepts in sociology make this effort worthwhile. Furthermore, it is the task of sociology to "sustain in regard to all elements of social life a spirit of unfettered, unsponsored inquiry, and the wisdom not to look elsewhere but to ourselves and not outside the discipline for this mandate" (Goffman 1983, 17). My study is guided by this dictum. I seek to argue neither for-or against clinical pharmacy or the physician extenders, only to understand fully those who are dominant by virtue of institutional authority and those who seek to alter these social arrangements.

The Social Context

The quest to remake the division of labor in health care is set against the social background of professional domination by medicine. This domination amounts not only to the power of medicine to control scarce resources but also to a widely shared belief that this profession should and can deal with matters of health and illness. In modern American society, expectations are such that we feel obliged to recognize the authority of medicine even when we are not compelled to seek the assistance of a physician every time we feel ill. There is a structure of expectations, constituting society's approval, that the medical profession is expert in matters of health and illness; members of society ought to use the services of doctors to solve these kinds of problems.

When this pattern of response to a problem exists, it can be said that the profession is institutionalized, making it almost a duty for the person in need of assistance to seek help from societally approved providers. An institution is defined as an organized way of providing some vital service. Once the legitimacy of an institution is established as the primary provider of important services—whether in matters of life and death, criminality, or safety—it can control those who will be allowed to perform these tasks. In contemporary society, the professions have gained control over their work environment and the requirements for entry into their fields; they have established ways of categorizing the problematic aspects of daily life and routine procedures for dealing with them. The professions, it can be said, have convinced society at large that they are capable of coping with the uncertainties of living. In an industrial society, which is based on a highly refined division of labor, they perform many coordinating and social-control activities by determining such questions as who is capable of working, who may own what property, the contractual obligations between consumers and suppliers or between management and labor, and how to build transportation networks or edifices that permit safe and easy access (Hughes 1967, 1–14).

In the area of knowledge about and use of medications, the profession of medicine established its position as the agent of control even before state licensing of physicians was widespread in the United States. By setting up the Council on Pharmacy and Chemistry in 1905, the American Medical Association (AMA) sought to lead the struggle against the sale of over-the-counter medications. In so doing, some physicians asserted quite simply that their advice was more important than the written material issued by the manufacturers of nostrums. The reformist spirit against patent medicines was made into association policy. No longer taking advertising in its journal for over-the-counter medications, the AMA, through its council, refused to approve any medication directly advertised to the public as useful to fight a disease. The AMA physicians sought to become the sole experts on diseases and on which medications were to be used to fight them. In establishing these rules and regulations, the AMA successfully won the right to become the institutional linkage between the patient and the drug manufacturer (Starr 1982, 131–133).

Once medicine's authority was established in these areas, the manufacturers of pharmaceuticals provided advertising revenues to the AMA, a resource used to create uniformity in outlook and social integration in medicine throughout the United States through strategic allocation. As Starr notes in his social history of American medicine, the AMA knew how to use its power to attain these goals.

> In 1912 the AMA set up a cooperative advertising bureau, which channeled advertisements to state medical journals. The bureau gave the AMA considerable financial leverage over the state medical

societies and helped bind the national association even more tightly together. Once again cultural authority was being converted into economic power and effective political organization. (Starr 1982, 134)

Later, following World War II, in response to the Truman administration's efforts to establish a national health insurance program, these same sources of funds were used to help the AMA keep its power.

> Organized medicine received large contributions from pharmaceutical firms to fight health insurance, in addition to the revenues from pharmaceutical advertising in AMA journals. The doctors received this support in part because of the strategic location they held in the marketing of drugs; their gatekeeping functions allowed them to collect a toll for use in political agitation. (Starr 1982, 288)

Starting from a more basic level, advocates of clinical pharmacy seek to alter the professional and public expectations held about pharmacy, thereby receiving recognition or cultural authority as experts on the uses and effects of drugs. This goal is certainly in line with the idea accepted in modern society that the expert is obliged to apply knowledge, not merely to understand the ways of the natural and social world. No matter how much pharmacists know about drugs, however, this knowledge and its uses must be recognized professionally and publicly, thereby making physicians and other health-care providers, and the general public, become obliged to listen to the advice proffered.

The role of the consulting expert, like any other role, is made up of expectations about the way individuals with specific social identifications (doctors, lawyers, pharmacists) will probably act in contact with others with identifications that are situationally specific (patients, clients). But there are also expectations held about what should be the proper beliefs and attitudes expressed by experts. Thus society requires that specific manners of expression go along with the procedures performed by the consulting expert. We might find it desirable that lawyers be aggressive, doctors thorough, and pharmacists careful.

What are the components of an expert's role? All roles have an instrumental side, oriented to getting certain things done, and an expressive side, representing the needs and preferences of collective life. Instrumental activities are means to achieve ends, while expressive activities are ends in themselves, generally promoting social solidarity. As ideas, these ways of looking at roles are useful because they help identify tensions that are built into successful and competent performance. The accomplishment of tasks, even when needed, can produce deep feelings of anger, which can interfere in these relationships.

Contact with patients requires the expression of a clinical attitude, not just providing advice. Patients sometimes voice dissatisfaction with the health-care expert when unexpected illnesses are uncovered, or, alternatively, when patients suspect that they are ill and feel that they are not being helped. Finally, any long-term service-receiving relationship is resented by both giver and receiver, since no final resolution of the problem appears in sight (Merton and Barber 1976). This situation would be particularly true for the chronically ill and disabled, or for people who have entered long-term psychotherapy. Sometimes it seems to both parties that the relationship has become an end in itself.

The clinical side of the work of an expert, then, has its uncertainties, some of which are built into the professional-client relationship. Still, many of these uncertainties are predictable in those professions that seek to apply knowledge on behalf of the client because there are shared situational expectations among those who seek and those who give help. Moreover, these relationships become institutionalized so that people know how to play these roles even before contact between clients and professionals are established.

The relationship between professional and client also forms a unit of social interdependency. The idea that the expert needs a client does not imply that the relationship is equal. Nor does this mean that because the client needs an expert, the relationship bestows greater power, prestige, and privilege on the giver of advice or performer of procedures; rather, these are advantages that are accumulated. That experts are able to accumulate these advantages stems from the justifications created to legitimate the relationship as well as from the actual assistance provided. It is the purpose of this book to explain the dynamics between rhetoric and action under the shadow of medicine.

References

Denzin, Norman K. 1972. "Incomplete professionalization: The case of pharmacy." In *Medical Men and Their Work: A Sociological Reader*, edited by Eliot Freidson and Judith Lorber, 55–64. Chicago: Aldine/Atherton.

Francke, Donald E. 1975. "Pharmacy in the year 2000." *Drug Intelligence and Clinical Pharmacy* 9: 454.

Goffman, Erving 1983. "The interaction order." *American Sociological Review* 48 (February): 1–17.

Hughes, Everett C. 1967. "Professions." In *The Professions in America*, edited by Kenneth S. Lynn, 1-14. Boston: Beacon Press.

Lamy, P.O. 1975. "Possible determinants of the practice of pharmacy in the year 2000." *Drug Intelligence and Clinical Pharmacy* 9: 426–429.

Merton, Robert K., and Elinor Barber 1976. "Sociological ambivalence." In Robert K. Merton, *Sociological Ambivalence and Other Essays*, 3-31. New York: Free Press.

Schwartz, M.A. 1975. "Educational needs for pharmacy practice in the year 2000." *Drug Intelligence and Clinical Pharmacy* 9: 447-451.

Starr, Paul 1982. *The Social Transformation of American Medicine: The Rise of a Sovereign Profession and the Making of a Vast Industry*. New York: Basic Books.

Tocqueville, Alexis de 1945. *Democracy in America*. Vol.2. Translated by Henry Reeve. New York: Vintage Books.

Zellmer, William A. 1976. "Patient package inserts." *American Journal of Hospital Pharmacy* 33: 535.

1 **Professions and Professionals in Modern Times**

Professions are both a very ancient and a modern phenomenon. Although found in ancient Greece and Rome, professions become a major normative force only in modern society; and it is useful to locate their ascendancy with the rise of industrial capitalism. In modern times we have learned to depend on professionals for many kinds of help. This dependency of clients on professionals marks a transition from a world in which family and clan were the major protectors of individuals against the irrationality and unpredictability of nature and society. Before the breakup of feudalism, the person without kinfolk or similar ties, had hardly any status in society and was virtually powerless. The ties that bound people together — kinship, fealty, and obedience — appeared to be fixed and frozen in time; and they provided assistance when needed.

The growth of cities challenged the hegemony of feudal ties and family supports when it came to dealing with problems such as health and safety. When strangers came together in large numbers, the encapsulated universe ended and new possibilities for careers open to talent arose. The rise of royal houses, representing the growth of the state, also meant that many professions, including medicine, architecture and law, would find patrons among the princes of Europe. Men of talent, like Leonardo da Vinci, could be useful in both peace and war, to solve recurring and emerging problems. Commoners still depended on folk healers, vernacular builders, and informal community advisers for help when they needed to go outside the family to solve their problems. Only with the rise of modern industry and the frequent and prolonged separations from community and kinfolk did the professional emerge in daily life.

An early nineteenth-century English novel, one of the first mystery stories in the language, revealed how the person alone could now stand a chance in making his or her way in this world. In Wilkie Collins's, *The Moonstone* (1944), the orphaned hero is able, with the help of various experts, to survive several attempts on his life. This exciting tale put the seal of approval on the use of outsiders to deal with the dangers of the world. The early development of such professions as law and medicine made it possible to manage on one's own.

Increasingly, in modern society, necessary tasks are accomplished through the use of experts who give advice and expect that advice to be followed. Relationships with experts are based on the belief in the efficacy of the provider's technology. Moreover, this technology is not a well-kept secret but is shared by those with similar social identities. Once it is accepted in society, the professional organization of work becomes both a way of getting things done and, most importantly for understanding the development of new professions, a model for the unorganized and less esteemed occupations. Others learn to control their members, their relations with clients, and their reputation, by emulating the sovereign professions. The rise of professional labor is one of the longest running trends of the past two hundred years (Larson 1977, 14–15).

The fledgling social sciences clearly found the professions and professionals a central part of modern life. The masters of nineteenth century sociological thought—Marx, Weber, and Durkheim—were keenly aware of the importance of users of knowledge to the development of modern societies. Each viewed the professions from his own theoretical perspective, producing the possibility of a rich, albeit blended, interpretation of their place and function in society. Marx saw experts doing the work of wielders of power—captains of the capitalist industrial enterprises that were changing the face of the world. Weber recognized the need to attribute a special status to experts in order to keep them going in their efforts to make the world more predictable, thereby encouraging the growth of rationality. Durkheim focused on the professional association—the community within the community—as the source of social identity and security in a world characterized by rampant individualism.

The professions remain the object of admiration today because of their moral independence and the perceived good that they do for others and for society. To promote the social benefits or functional value believed to come from the services rendered by the profession, societies in our times have encouraged professionals to form autonomous groups—not beholden to a patron or the public—to set forth the direction of advancement of knowledge or in applying it. This independence does not mean that professionals are outside the usual pressures faced by those who perform other occupational roles. Professionals, a corporate group, have a triangular relationship to clients, society, and to the profession itself.

Professionals, then, do not simply sell services, taking on all the other vendors in the marketplace in an open competition. Unquestionably, professions are highly organized occupations. They have a monopoly over a given set of tasks; and their clients are in an ambiguous position because they pay for services but do not possess the specialized knowledge necessary to evaluate fully the quality of the service actually or potentially provided. The playwright George Bernard Shaw once quipped that a profession is a conspiracy against the laity, meaning that its clients are vulnerable despite the fact that they are buyers. In addition, faith and trust play a substantial part in working with someone who provides services that are basically advisory. Moreover, by virtue of the nature of the problem—health, justice, safety—the clients need to have confidence in the professionals in whose hands they literally place their lives and sometimes their fortunes.

American sociology was quick to pay attention to the place of professions in a modern industrial society. It was one way to show how the norms of society could be so powerful that even when some people had superior knowledge, they would not use it to take advantage of others. Modern society was conceived of as being introjected to the extent that people complied with the norms even when not externally constrained to do so; and professional autonomy was considered a good thing because self-regulation as a form of social control was most compatible with an achievement-oriented society. Parsons (1939) held that the group life of the professions protects against exploitation of the public because all members of the profession internalize an ethical code that restrains them from taking advantage of the buyer. These scruples are supposed to keep professionals from acting unfairly toward clients. Control over the behavior of members of the profession is seen, according to this theory, to be best established through self-regulation, not through outside intervention. Peer review, another name for self-regulation, becomes the measure of all meaningful things in the profession because of the specialized quality of the work being performed. And this work is considered to be vital: Society has a compelling interest in seeing it get done, for individuals need to be cared for in order to feel part of society as well as to carry out or return to their full-time obligations. Therefore, the quality of life in society is affected by the widespread availability of professional services.

So far, the argument for professions in modern society suggests that the entity we call a profession is here for the benefit of all humanity, despite the great Anglo-Irish playwright's clever comment about conspiracies. Whether or not this is true, I am able to say with some confidence that the professions have convinced the society at large, and particularly elite groups, that they are capable of helping others to cope with the major uncertainties of living. Whether the functions they perform are real or imaginary, and whatever the cause—one based on society's innate wisdom in opting for autonomy for this unique work community or one that identifies the successful marketing of a service—the outcome has been the same. A few major professions—namely, law, medicine and engineering—have gained control over their work environments and the requirements for entry into the profession; they have established techniques for categorizing the problematic aspects of daily life and set up routine procedures for dealing with them. That experts have achieved this recognition or stature in society may be partly a result of the knowledge base of the profession and partly a result of the justifications created to encourage people to attribute to them dominance over certain vital services (Freidson 1970).

Note that I am presenting two contrasting views of society, embedded in these brief remarks about how professions acquire (1) power or command over scarce resources; and (2) status, or social honor, respect and admiration. In the first view, a kind of dialogue is carried on in which the role performed by the professional could be done in an exploitative or injurious fashion but instead will be performed correctly. In this view, the internalized commitments to the professional roles that some people play are taken as a constant or universal, and open competition or total state control of the professions is eschewed for the fully recognized benefits of peer control. In addition, the open market, wherein anyone can claim to have needed skills, is equally avoided.

This view reads almost like an interior monologue, one that reassures clients and the guardians of society that professional claims to effectiveness deserve ratification. The profession and its members receive admiration because they give services to a grateful society. The various parts of society, it appears, fit quite well. The deep commitment to the profession and its prospects prevents the knowledgeable doctor or lawyer from taking advantage of the unsuspecting client. Besides, these professionals are well trained technically and ethically, and *want* to be respected by their fellow professionals. In turn, peers will only honor the fellow professional who does not exploit clients. Most important, there is objective evidence that the technology professionals possess, made available only through in-depth professional training, is highly effective. Therefore there is little incentive to fool a client when it is evident that the solution designed by the professional is going to work. Like Voltaire's Dr. Pangloss, one feels lucky, knowing the above, to be in the best of all possible worlds.

In sum, the famous American sociologist Talcott Parsons basically saw society and its institutions as outside human construction or reconstruction, being both external and constraining. Professionals would not exploit clients because, by virtue of their training, a community orientation was introjected or internalized. Consequently, doctors, lawyers, and engineers want to do the right thing because it would be self-punishing for them not to do it. Socialization or the acquisition of knowledge, ability, and motivation, was perceived as appropriate to the role and effective. In addition, the knowledge available to them was effective and was rarely applied inappropriately, producing results that benefited the client. This knowledge-base was very valid and reliable, a fact known to all. Hence it was no mystery why society allowed these sovereign professions to regulate themselves: They had proven, clearly and objectively, their value to society. Known as the *functionalist* orientation, this view saw technical and professional recognition as the outcome of scientific progress rather than political efforts to stifle competition and gain advantages.

In 1970, Eliot Freidson's work on the application of knowledge and professional dominance suggested a more interactive and interpretive path toward professional autonomy. Like many other forms of social mobility, it was also a path to power and status. Starting with the assumptions that all occupations seek to control entry into them and have strong preferences as to the actual work environment where services are rendered, he was able to call into question the idea that medicine, or any other profession's, value to society was self-evident. In a carefully constructed argument, largely based on historical material, this sociologist of the professions proved that medicine received autonomy *prior* to demonstrating technical effectiveness. Clearly medicine made an effort to convince society that it should be self-regulating. The quest for autonomy and dominance is part of all drives for professionalization.

On another level of analysis, Freidson was able to demonstrate that medicine was perceived as a healing art even when it was of no value to the patient through proven therapies. In medical practice, he concluded, doctors were trained to find disease; and sometimes they found it when it was not there because the institutionalized norms pushed practitioners in that direction, making the sin of overlooking disease more serious than identifying it when it was not really there. Moreover, the very act of being treated, even with placebos, was shown to make people feel better.

Freidson was able to take apart Parsons's theory of the professions because Freidson was more widely read on the history of medicine, understood more about how impressions of success were created, even in the professions, and found support from other sociologists who specialized in the study of the professions. This powerful argument against the teleologic elements in functional analysis was supported by scholarly work on the legal profession, which showed that lawyers gained autonomy without a scientific body of knowledge (Rueschemeyer 1964). The linkage to state legislatures seemed especially warm to observers of the legal profession.

The theme of the need to gain the support of government for efforts at professionalization of a craft was echoed across the

Atlantic. Around the same time that Freidson's work on the profession of medicine was published, a British sociologist, Terrance Johnson, began to outline a methodology for the study of professions that focused on their relationships with those powerful credentialing bodies—national and state governments. Insofar as any government institution by law can grant a shelter from market competition, then they ought to be closely scrutinized to understand how one occupation gets sheltered and another does not. The granting or the removing of a professional monopoly on specific tasks are key events in the history of a profession. Consequently, Johnson suggests that the acquisition of power and status becomes a sequence of events that can be broken down and studied historically and comparatively, instead of focusing on the supposed generic elements of a professional versus a nonprofessional occupation.

In the United States, the work of political scientists examining the way in which supposed "regulatory agencies" such as the Food and Drug Administration or the Interstate Commerce Commission become coopted or heavily influenced by the representatives of the industries they are supposed to regulate should provide a clue to how this process works. In industries, as in professions and their licensing bodies, the regulators depend on information from the practitioners, making it likely that professions that get licensed are those in which outside knowledge is very limited. Every new profession, or one in transition, then works toward gaining independence from competitors and other constraints on their power. So far, there is much overlap with the work of Freidson.

By concentrating on the specific circumstances in which claims for professional status are made and ratified, Johnson (1972, 31) argued, we avoid the sterility of definition mongering and instead focus on two of the major empirical phenomena of our times: Group mobility through occupational upgrading, and the expansion of professionalism as a result of the growth of occupational group consciousness.

In this version of the story of the rise of professions, the occupational group's upward-mobility aspirations and the internal organization of the occupation become the key factors to be considered in any understanding of the power dimension in a profession's quest for autonomy. Johnson hypothesizes that since "occupational activities vary in the degree to which they give rise to a structure of uncertainty and in their potentialities for autonomy" (p. 43) we ought to look at these activities closely to locate the factors that help select out some occupations for self-regulation and not others. In a way, this appears to be the old functional-value argument coming back in a new guise. Is it not possible that an occupation can make claims for autonomy at any time because *new* uncertainties are now being faced and therefore more self-regulation needs to be granted? Moreover, what happens when the work of the profession becomes heavily predictable? Is autonomy eliminated and the occupation downgraded? These questions become crucial when we attempt to understand the arguments made by advocates for autonomy for those professions and practices that are attempting to gain greater responsibility in the division of labor in health care.

When we focus on uncertainties, they are usually translated into greater occupational responsibilities, that is, the need to exercise independent judgment (i.e., more authority). The way in which the occupation is organized and how the livelihoods of its members are realized are important in understanding which uncertainties are stressed. In the main, the focus of this book is on the new health-care practitioners who have come into being because of changes rendered by the transformation of American medicine into a high-technology, specialty-dominated profession. Sometimes the success of a dominant profession, based on the availability of new technologies and a movement toward greater specialization and managerial control, leaves great gaps in necessary preliminary services. With more years of education, fewer medical students want to practice family medicine (what used to be called *general practice*, a designation no longer recognized by medical associations and educational programs). Specialization draws students because it is where the action is in medicine; it yields greater rewards, both monetary and social (Silver 1976).

Similarly, the technological gains of the 1970s made adverse drug reactions a primary cause of hospitalization, creating a justification for a the new specialty called clinical pharmacy. Powerful medications had side effects, or when taken in combination or at the wrong dosage or wrong time of day, had a toxic effect on patients. Clinical pharmacy, it was claimed, could advise doctors and patients on how to avoid these consequences. The profession of medicine seemed to regard this task as one that did not require its attention. But these newly emerging health-care occupations raise all sorts of questions about how they will be regulated.

To what extent are these new health-care providers seeking greater autonomy and responsibility? Which practitioners, under what conditions, are able to make a drive for autonomy? Finally, how can the dominant profession differentially respond to these developments?

Occupations that are professionalizing are literally breaking out of their standardized or routine performance, and so require new kinds of control and direction in order to get others to understand what is going on. In a rare aphorism by a sociologist, Johnson observed that "a profession is not, then an occupation, but a means of controlling an occupation" (p. 45). The means of controlling a professionalized occupation is through credentials. This is a method of control based on standardization of the performer's education.

By establishing uniform educational requirements as a condition of entry into practice, the profession creates an entry barrier that sharply improves the market situation for existing practitioners. In his most recent opus, *Professional Powers* (1986), Freidson proffers the idea that credentialing serves to create "an occupational cartel which gains and preserves monopolistic control over the supply of a good or service in order to enhance the income of its members by protecting them from competition by others" (p. 63). Max Weber would have found this definition compatible with his conceptualization of the guild system of production during precapitalist epochs. The key difference between guilds and professionalized systems of control is the contemporary use of educational institutions as the source of ratification of membership in the occupational cartel.

Professions are, then, unique occupations that serve the powerful in society by solving other people's problems, but they do so at a cost: They are able to use labor-market shelters built around the higher education credentials they possess to gain some marginal power and a good deal of social status (Freidson 1986, 109). Thus their advice cannot easily be ignored because it is bought at a high price, even when the technology used has not proven to be effective. In sum, a profession may gain autonomy and control but it may not last forever. Change may occur, and the professional model of organization may become incompatible with some financial, technologic, and organizational developments.

The Idea of Sovereign Professions

In writing on the transformation of American medicine, Paul Starr (1982) uses the elegant expression "a sovereign profession" to refer to a time when medicine had enormous autonomy, an epoch that he regards as past. Both regulatory and market forces are creating new constraints on the practice of medicine. Under these twin pressures, medicine increasingly turns to ways of providing the same services at lower costs. To some extent, the delegation of tasks is nothing new in medicine, but the grounds for making the shift have changed greatly in the past twenty years.

Sovereign professions enjoy a special relationship with society, create unique bonds among those with credentials, and dominate the terms and conditions of their work with clients. In their efforts to focus exclusively on locating the nature of the client's problem and developing a solution to it, the professionals have always had the assistance of technical specialists or others with less depth or breadth to their education and training. It has usually been profitable for physicians, lawyers, and engineers to delegate tasks that are predictable and repetitive. The concern I have in this book is for the development of what are called physician extenders and clinical pharmacists, new practitioners in health care who have no cartel-like control over special tasks but seek special recognition and autonomy that would clearly distinguish them from others who assist the doctor. In addition, remuneration for these new tasks should be sufficient so that practitioners can give their practices their full attention. While much has been written about what tasks these new health-care practitioners will perform and how well they will perform them, there is scant theoretic guidance for understanding those who stand in the shadow of medicine and for predicting developments outside the technical sphere of their work.

Recently, a British sociologist, Gerald Larkin (1983), provided an unabashedly materialist view of the origin, emergence, and survival strategies of any occupation and its specific boundaries of competence. His approach focuses on the corporate group as both object to be buffeted about by forces outside its control and possessor of an internal survival code which presses it to become part of an existing division of labor. Unlike Johnson's work, Larkin's concern for the content of the craft is not found in his theoretical assumptions or postulates, nor are the specific assertions he makes directed to understanding occupational autonomy. It seems as if occupational autonomy is a chimera in his thinking about the material conditions surrounding occupations or, perhaps, an unachievable goal that occupational elites use to aspire to in order to gain some place in the division of labor.

The real struggle, for Larkin, is in the overall control of the division of labor, not over what actually goes on in the workplace or discussions and debates concerning who can perform what tasks most effectively and efficiently. He has studied three health-care occupations in Great Britain — ophthalmic opticians, radiologists and chiropodists (now designated *podiatrists* in the United States). Larkin's focus is exclusively on the nationally established councils, which are organized to regulate these different occupations. Outside this frame are such important considerations as the impact of technological advance, the changing education of medical doctors, and the way patient populations age.

The Professionalization of Medicine in a Historic Context

Medicine's autonomy and control over health care and other curing and caring occupations are recent events in the history of professions. Only in this century has the medical profession emerged as the socially defined repository of expertise necessary for the prevention, treatment, and amelioration of disease and illness. The current organization and delivery of health and medical care in the United States and elsewhere developed over a long period of small and sudden changes, reflecting changes in society generally and science and technology specifically. The institutional development of medicine and knowledge of disease is a tale of theoretical and practical advances in environmental control based on close observation and reasoned hypothesizing. In addition, the elimination of famines from some parts of the world, mainly where industrialization advanced most rapidly in the nineteenth century, made people more capable of withstanding infection. Medicine became more effective as a service when it had access to this secret ally—good nutrition. And so, ironically, treatment became the central foci of health care, even when preventive measures made it possible (McKeown 1965).

The medical expert became recognized as an important provider of support services in a society where labor's availability was becoming increasingly important. The division of labor grew in complexity, and the loss of labor time could result in the loss of production, distribution, and sales. When production on farms or in factories was based on a goal of selling in a remote market place and where transportation was needed for long-distance shipping, efficiency became important. Moreover, breaking down the work process into detailed and specialized labor also meant that later stages of production could not be accomplished unless earlier tasks were completed. Under these conditions, having workers away from their jobs, or, for that matter, the entrepreneur away from his or her place of business, was a liability. The division of labor, specialization, and the commercial way of life became recognized as an end in itself in the nineteenth century (Ure 1861). Thus social reproduction, or the production of the workforce, was a prerequisite for guaranteeing the formation of economic value.

More significantly, the great transformation to a capitalist system of production created severe dislocations of rural populations, alternatively coerced and attracted to urban industrial centers. Believing that poverty was the only way to get people to work (which justified low wages), nineteenth-century capitalists helped create conditions for the spread of disease, since adequate supplies of food, decent means of sanitation and a pure supply of water were beyond the means of factory workers. The middle classes and the very rich slowly became aware that they were creating the perfect environment for the spread of disease. Public health measures in Europe and the United States came about as a result of fear of contagion, since the respectable and the propertied could not remain completely apart from the poor (Greifinger and Sidel 1976, 10).

Medicine had socially integrative functions, as well as affecting public health. In the United States, the licensing of physicians was part of a general movement to create a professional and managerial class that would help promote entry of the immigrant working class into the fabric of American life, making sure that they would be productive members of the labor force and consumers of the products being produced in American factories and workshops (Ehrenreich and Ehrenreich 1977, 17). Medicine would become an "independent" force in modern society, working for the benefit of all. Physicians would acquire a special status as disinterested parties not directly in control of their patients' lives (in contrast to employers, for example), making physicians ideal agents for giving directives for living.

This moral authority was enhanced by a number of major reforms in medical education, spearheaded by the Carnegie Foundation's Flexner Report, an analysis of medical education released in 1910. Abraham Flexner, a social worker, saw medicine as one way of making life somewhat easier for the stressed poor. He envisioned licensed physicians, uniformly trained through a technical education, becoming public servants, sacrificing income to serve humanity. Proper medical education would train the physician to be oriented to the community, providing medical care free of charge or at moderate cost to those who otherwise could not afford it. As a political and social reformer during a time of great labor unrest marked by long and bitter strikes, Flexner was well aware that it was important to make workers feel that they were part of the American mainstream. Providing health services to the needy was one way to do this; at the same time, it ensured a healthy labor force.

Flexner was most concerned about the physical conditions in neighborhoods of large industrial and manufacturing cities along the Eastern Seaboard and in the Midwest. The major source of factory labor was from massive immigration to the United States from Eastern and Southern Europe. Overcrowding and inadequate ventilation and sunlight lead to high rates of tuberculosis and other diseases.

Efforts to improve living conditions had a political as well as an economic motive. Socialists and anarchists in America were making headway in convincing the new proletariat that conditions were intolerable and alterable. Reforms in medicine would hardly be sufficient to stop a quest for equality and dignity, but the Progressive era encouraged the development of a broad range of new and rejuvenated professions to help give the workingman the "square deal" he was looking for.

The Contemporary Context for Paramedical Professions

The Progressive era, which served as midwife to the development of modern professionalization, is also the historical bridge for the formation of a "new class" of professionals and managers called into being by capitalism to assist in the reproduction of capitalist social relationships. Unlike the proletariat, these semiautonomous professional workers produced the knowledge and information used in the production of commodities and in directing of the production system (Poulantzas 1975, 27).

Today, the masters of production and distribution (i.e., the leaders of capitalism) regard the health-care field in the United States as both necessary for the maintenance of a productive workforce, and as soaking up too much surplus capital that could be invested in production techniques which could make American industries of the United States more competitive with those of other nations. Lee Iacocca, the Chairman of Chrysler Corporation, has claimed that health benefits for workers negotiated through collective bargaining add to production costs and drive up the price of cars manufactured by American automakers.

Business leaders argue that America cannot be productive because the costs of social reproduction, are too high, causing a declining rate of profit. To corporate America, health care is at once a source of profits and a special interest that needs to be controlled and made more rational in its use of scarce resources. Capital in contemporary America sees health care as both a source of profits and a drag on productivity. The business community also notes the uneven way in which resources are distributed, a situation that has negative consequences for the larger corporations that pay for their employees health care. Smaller businesses are seen as getting off without providing health benefits to employees, who either pay for benefits themselves or receive uncompensated care from hospitals for major services. (These smaller enterprises will no longer be able to avoid paying for benefits if the Massachusetts model of universal health insurance is emulated in other states. See Sager 1988.)

The obvious success of American medicine in becoming the established deliverer of health-care services in the United States, driving out folk medicine, midwives and homeopathic healers, also required the development of the hospital as a workplace with a staff to whom repetitive tasks of care could be delegated. Within this legitimated order of service delivery, the physician became the manager of the health care team as well as the performer of procedures.

Using this unique form of self-organization—the professional association—medicine sought and received recognition as a sovereign profession. Within its direction, if not its outright control, grew nursing, pharmacy, and other *dependent and subservient* professions. These professions were in the shadow of medicine because they took their orders from doctors and received less deference from the public and the elites in American society. They had fewer opportunities to practice independent judgment as well as less responsibility for patient care, since they did not diagnose, develop treatment plans, or treat patients without supervision.

Nursing, pharmacy, and the newer physician-extender occupations (e.g., physician assistants) remain nested within the medical association and the physician dominated health-care system of the United States. By "nested," I mean more than the relational fact that physician extenders, makers of prescriptions, and nurturers of patients cannot perform certain tasks without the presence of doctors. I also want to stress that the parallel organizational structures found in related professional associations and licensures and journals are bounded by the profession of medicine and by its power and status in American society.

In turn, the unparalleled growth of health care in the United States, involving almost 12 percent of the gross national product (*GNP*), has called into being a broad-based health policy and planning sector. This specialty, referred to by Robert Alford (1972) as the "corporate rationalizers," has attempted to introduce limits to the growth of this major sector of the American economy. At best, it seeks to do this by redirecting resources within the health-care industry (e.g., shift utilization from inpatient to outpatient care). The growth of the new health-care practitioners is a direct result of the recognition of their contribution to the development of bureaucratic medicine.

References

Alford, Robert. 1972. "The political economy of health care: Dynamics without change." *Politics and Society* (Winter): 1–38.

Collins, Wilkie. 1944 [1868]. *The Moonstone*. New York: Doubleday.

Ehrenreich, Barbara, and John Ehrenreich. 1977. "The professional–managerial class." *Radical America* (March-April): 7–31.

Freidson, Eliot. 1970. *The Profession of Medicine*. New York: Dodd, Mead.
_____. 1986. *Professional Powers*. Chicago: University of Chicago Press.

Greifinger, Robert, and Victor Sidel. 1976. "American medicine: Charity begins at home." *Environment* 18: 7–18.

Johnson, Terrance. 1972. *Professions and Power*. London: Macmillan.

Larkin, Gerald. 1983. *Occupational Monopoly and Modern Medicine*. London: Tavistock.

Larson, Margalie Safatti. 1977. *The Rise of Professionalism*. Berkeley: University of California Press.

McKeown, Thomas. 1965. *The Modern Rise of Population*. New York: Academic Press.

Parsons, Talcott. 1939. *Essays in Sociology*. Glencoe, Illinois: Free Press.

Poulantzas, Nicolas. 1975. *Classes in Contemporary Capitalism*. New York: Humanities.

Rueschemeyer, D.1964. "Doctors and lawyers: A comment on the theory of the professions." *The Canadian Review of Sociology and Anthropology* 1: 17–30.

Sager, Alan. 1988. "Prices of Equitable Access: The New Massachusetts Health Insurance Law." *Hastings Center Report* (June/July): 21–25.

Silver, George. 1976. *A Spy in the House of Medicine*. Germantown, Md.: Aspen Systems.

Starr, Paul. 1982. *The Social Transformation of American Medicine: The Rise of a Sovereign Profession and the Making of a Vast Industry*. New York: Basic Books.

Ure, Andrew. 1861. *The Philosophy of Manufactures*. London: H.G. Bohn.

Chapter 2

The Growth of Bureaucratic Medicine

> Men make their own history, but they do not make
> it just as they please; they do not make it under cir-
> cumstances chosen by themselves, but under circum-
> stances directly found, given and transmitted from
> the past.
>
> — Karl Marx

The lineaments of modern health-care delivery can be found in the early history of the American hospital. We were out of the horse-and-buggy era in medicine long before doctors bought their first Model-T Ford. The bureaucratization of medicine started slowly, but even a century ago, milestones were established that indicated refinements in the division of labor and social organization of health care through functional and occupational specialization, the separation of decision making from the execution of routine tasks, and other features of complex organization that were identifiable in general hospitals. As early as 1872, hospitals developed specialized outpatient departments to care for particular diseases (Rosenberg 1987, 172). Even earlier, some hospitals created specialized laboratories to diagnose disease through analysis of patient specimens. Added to this was the increasingly capital-intensive technology to diagnose and treat, requiring its own supply of labor to make it work, without taking up the doctors' valuable clinical time.

Later, with improvements in nursing education and training, a further division of labor occurred as doctors delegated clinical tasks to this newly upgraded profession. Once the refuge of the disrespectable, nursing, through educational reforms, increasingly attracted able and ambitious women, producing the seeds of a continuous struggle that was to continue both within their ranks and with medicine (Rosenberg 1987, 236). To some extent, the same struggle is being reproduced now that the profession of medicine has called into being physician assistants and nurse practitioners.

The hospital became the centerpiece in the health delivery system in which we have such abiding faith. As a complex organization, it is a tool to help reproduce the society by curing or at least by producing palliative assistance. What the hospital needed was a linkage to the marketplace, since it was originally a vehicle for the spread of social welfare and for care of the unwanted and unloved. Charles Rosenberg (1987) observed that "the late twentieth-century hospital already existed in embryo, waiting only the nutrients of third-party payment, government involvement, technological change, and general economic growth to stimulate a rapid and in some ways hypertrophied development" (p.349).

The baby not only was brought to term but grew to become the model for how all medicine should conduct its practice. The hospital captured medicine, giving it an aura and respect it never had before. The overspecialization, extreme dependence on hospital care, testing, and increasingly higher remuneration and veneration made culture heroes out of most doctors in private practice. Along with this improvement in status in the eyes of the public came new problems of management in the day-to-day delivery of inpatient care, creating solutions that became pathways for the development of practitioners with new responsibilities and opportunities to use clinical judgment.

New Practitioners, New Relationships

In the nineteenth century, community notables (mainly business and factory owners) and members of religious orders started hospitals to create an orderly and predictable world. Physicians used hospitals more to learn about disease than to treat patients. In many instances, doctors maintained direct contact with patients throughout their illnesses, particularly if patients were cared for at home by a family that could provide the necessary attention. Sometimes families specialized in caring for individuals who had no kin or were in unusual circumstances, such as a traveler who became ill in a foreign place.

The links between medicine and nursing, to name the profession of the most direct clinical assistant to the doctor, were inconsistent until certain organizational and technological developments occurred in the second half of the nineteenth century, when war made nursing a necessary component of hospital care. Nurses, under the direction of Florence Nightingale (in the Crimean War) and Clara Barton (in the American Civil War), proved their worth in saving lives. Treating the wounded at or near the battlefield could not have been undertaken without disciplined nurses who could take over some of the doctor's tasks.

Prior to these events, nursing was the province of female members of religious orders and, sometimes, secular organizations. The new form of health care resembled a military organization. Orders were followed in a disciplined way, and specific tasks were assigned to clearly identified positions in a division of labor. Doctors and nurses were guided by explicitly stated duties, set down in written rules, and their positions were hierarchically organized so that decision making and information gathering — the procedures of diagnosis and treatment — were clearly in the hands of the physicians. This hierarchical organization was evident in the respect nurses accorded to doctors, even to standing up whenever a doctor entered a room.

A social organization such as this is based on coordinating the efforts of various specialists. The solution to the task of dealing with hundreds or even thousands of wounded followed procedures that have come to be known as bureaucracy. Given the magnitude and pervasiveness of the problem, the application of bureaucracy to wartime health care was necessary.

During the late nineteenth and early twentieth centuries, technological advances made possible more precise diagnoses and treatment and standard surgical procedures. The invention of the X-ray machine meant that the source of some disorders could be located and that physicians could see bones that were broken or in the process of healing. Anesthesia made surgery more manageable, while techniques established to prevent sepsis (the infection of wounds during and after surgery) made it possible to save lives that previously would have been lost.

New technology made specialization and coordination even more important than it had been in the past. Physicians became dependent on the hospital as a workshop. The centralized location of facilities and equipment meant that several doctors could use them when needed. The availability of a nursing staff also made daily care more predictable. A pool of paying patients (i.e., a market) could be directed to a hospital, where physicians knew in advance that their orders for patient care would be followed.

The organization of a hospital along bureaucratic lines may appear to result from the increase in the number of patient beds. Size, however, does not fully explain the development of formal organizational characteristics, such as written rules, specifically designated times and groups for policy discussions, and job descriptions at all levels. Starkweather (1970) found that complexity of organization encouraged the development of formal channels of communication, agreement on common purpose, and specifications of jobs and authority. In his study of 704 general hospitals, "size, identified independently from complexity was not found to influence formal organization mechanisms significantly" (p.338).

Complexity has led acute-care hospitals to adopt a team approach, a reorganization of the formal relationships found in the bureaucratic structure of hospitals. Making complicated decisions about therapy requires enormous inputs of information about the patient's condition, behavior, and previous health history and gaining the cooperation and compliance of those involved in the treatment plan. It is assumed that professionals who help develop the plan will be more encouraged to carry it out than those who are simply told what to do.

The team creates a form of involvement as well as peer pressure. A major assumption of the idea of a health-care team is that a patient's problems can be best handled by those directly involved with the patient on a regular basis. While members of the health-care team are responsible to a unit manager or a team leader, decisions must often be made quickly and on the basis of full information about the patient. As Beckhard (1972) found, "'ownership' in decisions goes far toward effective implementation" (p. 305–6).

The desire to reduce the cost of medical care by reducing hospital admissions and long stays has been another factor in fostering the team approach. The growth of middle-level practitioners is based on providing outpatient or ambulatory care. With fewer cases of acute illness and more of chronic illness, there has been more concern with the management of illness. As a result, monitoring patients has become a long-term and important ongoing task. Other tasks delegated by physicians involve primary care for children (known as well-baby visits) and the physical examination of adults where standardized procedures exist. Since physicians do not always observe the patient or the work performed by the middle-level practitioner, a team approach allows information to be shared among all team members. Team meetings become a forum for the dissemination of information and the development of a treatment plan.

New Demands and Health Care Planning

With increasing demand for services in the 1960s, brought about by public financing of medical care for the elderly and the indigent in the Medicare and Medicaid programs, there was suddenly a lack of physicians, particularly in the poorer rural and inner-city areas of the United States. Demand did not grow as the population expanded, it grew more rapidly because demand is affected by the age composition of the population more than by any other factor. The volume of demand in the health-care field is elastic, driven by the availability of third-party financing. No sicker than in the past, the public now saw the use of doctors as part of a decent way of life rather than something to be done with caution or only in serious illnesses. By the 1970s, physicians were making considerable incomes from private practice, and still there were not enough of them to go around.

Twenty years ago, medical and health planners, and some ordinary citizens as well, were very concerned about the shortage of physicians in the United States. In 1960, there were only 14 physicians for every 10,000 people in the population, and there was enormous regional variability in the distribution of these medical and osteopathic doctors. By 1970, the situation had improved only slightly; there were 15.6 physicians for the same 10,000 Americans, hardly an enormous increase during a turbulent decade that saw the initiation of Medicare and Medicaid (National Center for Health Statistics 1985, 106).

These programs radically expanded the market for medical care in the United States.

Moreover, the physician shortage was particularly devastating in the area of primary care since most medical students were deciding to become specialists. General practice was being relegated to the scrap heap, along with the house call and the direct payment to the doctor for services rendered. Critics began to recognize a strange paradox in American health care: We technologically advanced medicine to deal with serious threats to life or functioning, but it was hard to find doctors to do day-to-day prevention, health education (now called health promotion), and early treatment of minor (and even serious) maladies.

Specialists in health policy and planning—the corporate rationalizers—decided to do something about this maldistribution of a necessary service. Policymakers and planners were found mainly in the various bureaus of the Department of Health and Human Services (known at that time as the Department of Health, Education, and Welfare); in a few centers or institutes designed to give theoreticians the leisure to solve important practical problems, or in the schools of public health, both at elite private medical colleges with substantial endowments and the more progressive state medical schools. They were concerned with finding ways of delivering the much needed services involved in primary care but without using the overtrained, expensive, and overworked physicians to do it. These planners and policymakers began to invent professions to assist the doctor—not merely to do the boring and repetitive tasks that made up the bulk of nursing but to act more as a substitute for the doctor. Such professionals would make decisions on their own, would carry their own patient panels, and would be able to use their abilities to help patients face the uncertainties of living. In other words, the doctor would be able to delegate tasks of some complexity, not merely the unwanted and highly routinized tasks delegated to hospital nursing staffs or the clerical tasks given over to office personnel.

A second source of concern for the corporate rationalizers was the enormous cost and waste of resources when people were admitted to hospitals unnecessarily because the services they required were not available on an outpatient basis or their physician did not have the time to orchestrate and manage diagnostic testing because there was no health practitioner in the office-based practice to arrange for these tests. Waste of resources was also defined by these planners as overly long hospitalizations because there was no one to monitor the patient following discharge. Therefore, hospitalization was perceived as occurring too frequently and with an average length of stay that was not supportable, given the nature of the conditions and/or the wide variation in length of stay associated with treatment of the same condition.

The growth of the hospital as the major organizational form for delivering health care accounts, at least in part, for rising service costs. Aside from inflation and population growth during the past 30 years, increased utilization of short-term or general hospitals has spurred the rise in costs, with patient days in hospitals per 1,000 in the population increased from 1,072 in 1956 to 1,194 in 1973 (Cambridge Research Institute [CRI] 1975, 163). In 1974, hospital care accounted for 39 percent of national health expenditures (CRI 1975, 155). Total expenses for nonfederal short-term hospitals rose from $5.6 million in 1960 to $28.5 million in 1973, a five-fold multiplication of costs. The rate of increase in the post-Medicare/Medicaid period was far higher than from 1960 to 1968 (CRI 1975, 162). With federal, state, and local governments bearing 39.6 percent of the costs of all expenditures in 1974, planners became increasingly concerned about ways to reduce the need for hospitalization.

If medical home-care services could be delivered by a less expensive source than the medical doctor, it was reasoned, patients could go home earlier, thus saving billions of dollars in hospital days as well as promoting a return to family and community. Furthermore, by monitoring patients during recovery at home, the new practitioners could prevent rehospitalization and reduce the adverse psychological consequences of separation from the family, particularly for children. Clearly, there were cost savings involved if these new health providers could be trained and used to reduce the medical and hospital bill in the United States.

Designated middle-level health-care practitioners, these providers of care extend the physician's competence beyond direct contact with patients. Specific titles for these positions vary, with the two most popular being physician assistant and nurse practitioner. Most training programs (but not all) focus on preparing people to assist physicians in primary care, the first point of contact between patients and the health-care delivery system.

In the division of labor in health care, nurses for many years have been given routine tasks that physicians found relatively simple but time-consuming. Many of the four-year baccalaureate degree programs for student nurses are based on being able to perform such tasks as taking blood pressure, administering intravenous feedings, and reading electrocardiogram machines. In fact, if a nurse could not quickly read a vital-life-sign indicator and take immediate action, many intensive care units could not have been established. The new roles of physician extenders simply follows an established trend, but creates interesting possibilities.

The time seemed right in the middle of the 1960s to try new things, but advocates of similar plans in the past have met with considerable opposition, sometimes from surprising sources. In 1927, a physician named Alfred Worcester wrote a book that advocated

> advanced training to enable the nurse to become the doctor's assistant in medical tasks. Because nursing education and nursing service would be controlled by doctors, his plans were opposed by nursing leaders representing both the Nightingale and professional orientation. Nor did he get the support of the medical profession since he worked at a time when doctors did not feel a great need to delegate medical tasks; he might have gotten their support today. (Glazer 1966, 27–8)

Founders of the first training programs for physician assistants and nurse practitioners, created at Duke University Medical School in 1965, were convinced that physicians had been too highly trained to do routine medical tasks. These new roles were created in order to utilize the skills of physicians appropriately and cut the costs of health-care delivery. Since nurse practitioners and physicians assistants work alongside the doctor, the general title of *physician associate* will be used here to refer to both roles.

Duke University pioneered the promotion of both kinds of physician associates but is best known for its two-year training courses for physician assistants; by 1975, there were eighty four training programs for physician assistants in the United States (CRI 1975, 371). In these early days, students usually had two to four years of college and some previous health-care experience. Recruitment from former military medical corpsmen and hospital nurses took place, although the tendency at that time was for males to be tracked in physician associate programs and women into nurse practitioner training programs because of the traditional gender associations.

The cost of training a physician associate for one year was as much as a year of medical school in these pioneering programs. However, the overall length of training was less than for a physician (CRI 1975, 376). In addition, salaries were (and still are) much lower for physician associates than for medical doctors (Silver 1976, 97). The belief of the "corporate rationalizers" was that billing for the physician associates' services would be lower because of the lower cost of education. But the management and supervision by physicians put these extenders of care on a par with physicians as far as fees were concerned. Doctors collected the same amount from patients whether they personally delivered the service or it was provided by a surrogate. And of late, hospitals and health maintenance organizations (HMOs) are starting to employ new health practitioners as a cost-reducing feature of running programs.

Not all doctors immediately endorsed the new providers. In spite of the physician shortage, some M.D.s saw the new health-care practitioners as potential competitors rather than ways to expand their practices. Nevertheless, early studies were enthusiastic. A 75 percent increase in the number of patients was reported by incorporating a physician assistant in a single practice, with no reduction in the quality of care (Cihlar 1975, 54).

In some cases, physician associates are utilized to provide care in isolated or impoverished areas of the country where few physicians are found. But working under the condition of low availability of physicians does not provide the necessary consultation required to provide adequate medical care. Most new health practitioners work in private group practices or in clinics where close contact with physicians is possible. By the middle of the 1970s, a high proportion (one-third) of physician assistants were practicing in non-urban areas, compared to only 13 percent of all physicians (Institute of Medicine 1978).

The 1980s have seen an enormous investment of private capital into the health-care delivery system. At one time confined to the pharmaceutical industry, investors now have encouraged the development of multihospital systems owned by large corporations, some with worldwide holdings. This same decade has also witnessed the growing importance of purchasers of health care — corporations and collective buyers — aiming to do the unheard of in this field: to "negotiate price, method of payment, scope of services and guarantees to render all services for a preestablished price per patient" (Light 1986, 527). Employers now attempt to save money for health benefits for employees by steering them to preferred provider organizations (PPOs), caregivers that charge the self-insured corporation less than if employees went to just any provider in the community. To encourage utilization, employers offer those covered by these plans a lower deductible or copayment if they use a provider that belongs to the plan. Managers of these plans may consider using physician associates to keep their costs down and pass on the savings to self-insured corporations.

A major problem for the hospitals, agencies, and prepaid health service groups (HMOs) is the cost of delivery of services. Health care is both a capital-intensive field (since equipment is expensive and constantly is upgraded) and a labor-intensive one (since patients require a great deal of attention). Consequently, managers of both inpatient and outpatient delivery systems are eager to substitute for expensive and scarce medical doctors, wherever possible. Most important, the charges for a procedure rendered by physician associates are the same as for a physician, but the costs in the form of salaries are far lower.

These developments should help slow the rise in the cost of health care. Recently, a central issue in several major strikes was a demand by management to have employees pay for more of the costs of their families' health care (e.g., Pittston, NYNEX).

Cost Containment and Task Shifting

The new health practitioner becomes especially valuable during periods of cost consciousness, regardless of whether an organization is profit making or nonprofit. Task shifting of primary-care functions to physician associates makes financial sense whether the bottom line is profit or allocation of funds for other providers.

Task shifting involves not only replacement of physicians in primary care with new health practitioners but using them to keep people well or, in the case of prepaid programs, getting them to stay out of hospitals. In a system where a fixed charge for the entire year is paid on a per capita basis, the providers who give care in a way that is mindful of the budget limitations of the program are preferred to those who order unnecessary tests and often hospitalize their patients. A balance must be struck between the needs of the patient and the capacity of the organization to take care of every minor problem that comes up.

Managers of HMOs and hospitals, which must live under the prospective payment system introduced to reimburse hospitals for Medicare patients, have a lot in common. They both need to find physicians who can keep expenses down while getting patients well in a shorter period of time than in the past. Prospective payment provides hospitals with a fixed sum for treating patients with similar diagnoses, regardless of difference in treatment costs. Thus the charges for patients who have hernia repairs will be the same in every hospital even if patients stay fewer or more days than the average length of stay. Known as diagnosis-related groups (DRGs), the 470 groups of diseases have calculated average charges associated with them. Under this financing system, hospitals are paid a fixed sum based on the case mix they had in previous years.

Cost-conscious managers will not only attempt to avoid unnecessary treatments once a patient is hospitalized but also will seek to use cost-effective labor to deliver services. The use of new health practitioners in hospitals is limited at this time. Yet there are signs that they can be used to replace surgical residents when the hospital makes a policy decision *not* to train any more of those specialists in an already overcrowded field.

The Crisis in Pharmacy

Pharmacy provides a real challenge to a sociological analysis of the professions. Rarely have we considered how, and under what conditions, an established profession seeks to change its position within a single industry. A profession can be affected by various developments: A new technology can take away functions from established practitioners; it can find new markets and organizational structures, delegating tasks to lesser-trained occupations; and other occupations may try to encroach on it by increasing educational requirements and adopting a code of ethics.

I would predict that, under these conditions, new elites will emerge who try to redirect the profession toward solutions that will help it maintain its power and status, perhaps even enhance them. It will be interesting to see what kind of response these new leaders will receive, internal to the profession and from other professions with which a division of labor is shared.

The case of reprofessionalization in pharmacy provides an opportunity to learn more about the interactive and contextual nature of the development of the professions in the shadow of medicine. The development of clinical pharmacy is not sponsored by the medical societies and associations of the United States, nor is it part of the work of the corporate rationalists at the Department of Health and Human Services or at the schools of public health.

Still, there is clearly a need for a theoretically driven examination of the structural changes that have produced an effort on the part of some segments of pharmacy to respond in a positive way to this crisis. The purpose of this analysis is to make predictions about the tendencies of particular beliefs or solutions to the general problem of the field to produce role stability. Other sociologists of professions find it useful to focus on "concrete occupational strategies as well as wider social forces and arrangements of power" (Klegon 1978, 259–283). Can we consider the clinical pharmacy movement as a distinct social strategy for dealing with critical change within the industry and not just a way of technical problem solving? How is it that an effort is being made within pharmacy to upgrade its power and status? What specific factors need to be identified that can account for this movement?

Some sociologists simply see the movement to clinical pharmacy as a way to deal with drug iatrogenesis as a social problem. Claiming that clinical pharmacy was developed to reduce instances of adverse drug effects due to prescription errors by physicians, the sociologists sympathetic to its claims also legitimate clinical pharmacy, giving it a social purpose (Broadhead and Facchinetti 1985, 425). While the lines between advocacy and analysis need not always be drawn sharply, some supporters seem to select out a "patient-focused" and altruistic role for pharmacists to play while ignoring the larger historic developments that have shaped the profession.

Few empirical studies of professions can guide this inquiry. The changing division of labor, technology, social organization, and economic support of the health professions have received little investigation by sociologists of professions. Kronus (1976) has examined the historic evolution of pharmacy and medicine in the differing social contexts of nineteenth century England and the United States. Informal efforts by apothecaries in England to attend to the health-care needs of the middle-class client population were rewarded by social support, eventually culminating in the evolution of this role into the medical general practitioner. In contrast, pharmacists in the United States were relegated to technical-support roles to medicine because the profession of medicine was successful in controlling health-care delivery. Using a more quantitative approach, Begun and Feldman (1981) examined the political activities of optometrists in four states with widely different economic, political and social characteristics in their study of how this profession was and was not successful in limiting competition.

One segment of pharmacists advocates turning their profession in a clinical direction. The better educated in the field are capable of assuming new responsibilities involving the performance of qualitatively different roles from those performed by pharmacists in the past. The clinically minded see themselves as possessing knowledge that directly benefits patients and performing services that deserve respect from patients and physicians.

This movement in pharmacy cannot be understood apart from developments in health care that have imposed greater uniformity and predictability in the work situation of the pharmacist, mainly through increased bureaucratic organization and specialization. The movement toward reprofessionalization is a reaction to these changes.

The specter haunting the profession of pharmacy is manifest in the fear of displacement and a downgrading of the craft. This concern is strikingly similar to fears expressed by English artisans in the late eighteenth century when they were faced with the rise of the factory system (Thompson 1963). The honorable craft of pharmacy now faces a loss of power and control over scarce resources, including the utilization of learned skills, and a loss of status and social approval.

The field of pharmacy offers an excellent contrast to the emergence of the new health-care practitioners. The profession's reaction to the stress of new developments provides the background to the clinical aspirations of some pharmacists. Elites in pharmacy advocate reprofessionalization but are met with resistance within and outside the field. The goal of upgrading pharmacy to the level of a clinical profession involves the acquisition of qualitatively different roles from those performed by members of the profession in the past. Simply to view pharmacy as smoothly changing from craft to profession ignores the new consciousness of members of the profession who see themselves as clinicians. For example, they see a need for intervening on patients' behalf because of their recognition that adverse drug interactions can lead to death and are one of the ten leading causes of hospitalization. The pharmacist, by virtue of careful recordkeeping on patients and a knowledge of drug effects, would be able to warn patients and (physicians) when a drug therapy is prescribed that can adversely interact with a drug already being taken by a patient. The new practice is defined by its advocates as "the application of pharmaceutical service emphasizing integration and coordination of the patient's total drug regimen, using all available means to achieve maximum effectiveness and safety of drug therapy in the context of the patient's total environment" (Provost 1972, 77).

Justification for the new practice is further expressed in the priorities of Jere E. Goyan (Lyons 1979), a former head of the

Food and Drug Administration and a former dean of a college of pharmacy: "We need to devote more time to . . . the effect that as many as eight different drugs taken concurrently might have on those persons who might be taking them all."

Nevertheless, recognition of the need to keep drug profiles on patients does not automatically produce appropriate clinical behavior by pharmacists. Dr. Goyan conceded that clinical pharmacy was far from standard practice in every community or hospital pharmacy. His admission that there is still a "long way to go" before all pharmacists are clinicians reveals some of the built-in tensions in the profession (Lyons 1979). The clinical pharmacy advocate, in reinventing pharmacy, is seeking to change the knowledge, ability, and motivation of pharmacists and convince outsiders (e.g., physicians and hospital administrators) that pharmacists should be allowed to consult with patients and physicians. Having complete control over entry into the profession — physicians do not sit on state pharmacy licensing boards — has been an insufficient basis for acquiring new responsibilities.

Medicine is not the only source of resistance. Clinically oriented members of the profession are also critical of the lack of unity in pharmacy. They note that community and hospital pharmacists have few common professional interests, that many older pharmacists show no interest in acquiring new knowledge and responsibilities, and there is a great deal of competition between community pharmacies. Further, the clinically oriented find that physicians and patients do not sufficiently respect pharmacy, claiming that the entire profession is judged by its worst aspects — high drug prices, steering patients to over-the-counter drugs, lavish gifts to physicians and filling illegal prescriptions.

Given the intense competition engendered by the capitalization of pharmacy through chain stores and the success of mass-production techniques in the manufacture of pharmaceutical products, additional consequences are inevitable for the field.

Conflicting views on the place of pharmacy in the health-care delivery system reflect macrocosmic changes — new technology, social organization, and division of labor — on the functions of the profession. The remainder of this chapter examines the origins of this crisis in pharmacy.

Origins of the Crisis

The traditional organization of the field permitted pharmacists to combine professional and business orientations (Denzin 1968; Mechanic 1970; Kronus 1975). The community locations of retail pharmacies allowed the sale of patent medicines and sundries as well as filling prescriptions. Unlike physicians, who are constrained by the ongoing character of their relationships with patients, pharmacists could devote considerable time to building up the business part of their practice. This produced a mixed image of the pharmacist and the community pharmacy ("the drug store") as half profession, half business—an image rejected by faculties of colleges of pharmacy, who view themselves and their recent graduates as militant upholders of professionalization, combining enthusiasm for change with challenges to existing social arrangements in community and hospital pharmacies.

This characterization of the field of pharmacy is supported by editorials and articles in pharmacy journals and interviews with practicing pharmacists. Hospital pharmacists are perceived as well suited to the role of change agent (Kormel 1978). Pharmacists run special clinics in hospitals to increase the rate of patient compliance with physician's medication regimens (Schneider and Cable 1978). Pharmacy is seen as "changing from a response oriented to an active, participatory system" (Lamy 1978, 1).

The reaction of physicians and other health-care providers to the changing role of the pharmacist is of great concern to those who advocate change. They make assessments of physicians' attitudes toward pharmacists as drug information consultants (Nelson, Meinhold and Hutchinson 1971; Adamcik and others 1986). The drug prescribing patterns of physicians are also studied by pharmacists concerned with adverse drug effects (Christensen and Bush 1981). Finally, new skills needed for pharmacists to play clinical roles, such as interviewing techniques, are considered to be important in establishing the right to play these roles (Love and others 1978).

Five structural changes in the organization and delivery of pharmaceutical services are discussed in the remainder of this section. They have encouraged the movement within pharmacy to adopt clinical roles. These factors are threats to the power and status of pharmacists, and I believe that clinical pharmacy is a collective response to occupational displacement.

The Decline of the Community Pharmacy

There has been a reduction in the number of small retail pharmacies in the United States, as large "discount" drug stores replace pharmacist-owned establishments. Independent owners who operated pharmacies found this arrangement a satisfactory way of earning a livelihood, one that even provided opportunities for employing other pharmacists. But as early as 1968, observers of the field noted that "aggressive chain operators are dispensing prescriptions at lower cost to the patient" [and] these lower charges are possible due to purchase economies and increased promotion of the prescription department" (Knapp and Knapp 1968). According to the National Association of Boards of Pharmacy (1987–1988), although data are missing from twenty-two states, one out of every five pharmacies in the United States in 1986 was part of a chain. Moreover, the 1986–1987 report of the American Association of Colleges of Pharmacy found that 43 percent of their graduates went to chain pharmacies, a trend that is expected to continue.

Like many other small businesses, independent community pharmacies were hurt by court decisions in the 1960s that declared fair trade agreements as a constraint on trade. The National Association of Retail Druggists, organized in 1898, led the struggle for protective state legislation on pricing. Consequently, the proliferation of chain stores that gave discounts on prescriptions and sundries was checked (Smith and Knapp 1976). But state courts declared some fair-trade agreements with manufacturers to set minimum prices illegal, and as a result, large discount drug outlets have grown over the past twenty years. "From 1964 to 1984 alone, the number of chain stores grew by 246 percent, while the number of independents dropped by 31 percent, according to a study by Jean Paul Gagnon, professor of pharmacy administration at the University of North Carolina" (Holcomb 1988, 60). Evidence of this kind suggests a diminution of opportunities for the pharmacist who wants the autonomy that comes with ownership, "to be my own boss."

Pharmacy's strong roots in entrepreneurial activities is also reflected in the lack of appeal that purely professional associations have had for pharmacists, as compared to physicians and dentists. As of 1987, among the 116,500 practicing pharmacists in the United States, only 25 percent belonged to the broad umbrella organization, the American Pharmaceutical Association.

The need for professional membership is weak in community pharmacy where day-to-day interaction with other professionals is infrequent. Merton (1958) has hypothesized that one function of a professional association is to reduce power and status differences that occur in the workplace and make communication among various professional associations possible, perhaps even convincing other professions that high standards of training and performance are ensured. Consequently, in hospital pharmacy, a higher percentage of potentially eligible members (i.e., pharmacists who work in hospitals) belong to the American Society of Hospital Pharmacists. In 1975, the potential-to-actual membership rate was over 85 percent (Smith and Knapp 1976, 120).

Automation

Pharmacy is a field threatened by automation, both in the manufacture of drugs and their dispensing in hospitals and nursing homes. Mechanic (1970) noted that pharmacy faced a crisis of purpose brought about when manufactured drug combinations made compounding unnecessary. Today, some state licensing examinations for pharmacists have eliminated questions on compounding techniques. As a result of this development in technology, the pharmacist provides consumers with a service in which skill related to product formulation is not needed.

The enormous expansion of hospitals and nursing homes has created many employment opportunities in pharmacy, but they hardly require the performance of traditional crafts. In the future, even the traditional role of dispensing medication may be limited, since automated dispensing and packaging is already being used to fill individualized prescriptions for hospitalized patients. The techniques combine computerized prescriptions with vending- machine-like equipment that can be programmed;

licensed pharmacists are not needed to perform these tasks. Pharmacy technicians and assistants can tend these machines under the supervision of a single licensed pharmacist. This separation of decision making from the performance of routine tasks takes place in the design of work and work settings, a process often noted in American industry (Braverman 1972).

Physician Extenders

Some of the motivation for moving in a clinical direction stems from feelings that status decline results from the increased responsibilities of nurses and the invention of mid-level health care practitioners — providers who were once seen as socially and educational inferiors to pharmacists. The development of middle-level health-care provider roles, such as physician assistants and nurse practitioners, has created a great deal of interest on the part of pharmacists in upgrading their responsibility and authority in hospitals. Pharmacists would like to receive more recognition for the work they do as medication-control agents, educators of other health-care providers, and monitors of patient compliance with physician-ordered prescriptions. While demanding clear delegation of these responsibilities, hospital pharmacists are also experiencing a loss of status brought about by technological displacement and exacerbated by new practices and regulations that permit nurse practitioners to diagnose and prescribe for minor illnesses (under the standing orders written by a physician). Thus, pharmacists now take orders from providers they may regard as not well trained. Furthermore, the close clinical contact between nurse practitioners (or physician assistants) and both patients and physicians is a source of envy for the pharmacist. Advocates of an expanded role for pharmacists speak of the acquisition of clinical responsibilities and the right to charge a fee for the service, both in hospital and community practices (Provost 1972, 235; Anonymous 1973, 23). Currently, only Florida and the state of Washington permit pharmacists to prescribe, and to charge for writing the prescription; only permission extends to a limited number of medicines in a limited number of categories involving only minor illnesses (National Association of Boards of Pharmacy 1987–1988).

New Patterns of Recruitment

Recent attrition of vocational opportunity in the natural sciences, particularly in university and college research and teaching positions, may have attracted more academically minded students to the profession of pharmacy. Since pharmacy training in the United States is now part of five- and sometimes six-year baccalaureate degree programs, the field is more interesting to students who wish a scientific education with some potential for following a research career. Although in the past pharmacists interested in academic careers or opportunities to do research in commercial laboratories acquired Ph.D. degrees, the newly created Pharm.D. degree reflects efforts to upgrade the field both educationally and clinically. The new degree makes pharmacy a field in which people have received advanced training *as* pharmacists, combining scholarly potential with immediate economic opportunity. Compared to vocational opportunities for biologists and chemists, recent pharmacy graduates who acquire state licenses have easily found employment. Pharmacy schools report that jobs are readily available for their students, that enrollments are increasing after a decline in the early 1980s, that almost 55 percent of their undergraduates are women, and that starting salaries are impressive, particularly in the chains (Glaser 1987; Anonymous 1987, 15–16).

Communication among Pharmacists

The generalized fear among pharmacists of being displaced would not have been possible if the disgruntled had not been able to find out that their dissatisfaction was shared with others. The expansion of the field of pharmacy depends on the continued use of drugs in treatment, making for growth not only in chain pharmacies but in hospital and nursing home pharmacies as well; the number of hospital pharmacists doubled in the 1970s (Zellmer 1979, 36). Today, there is far more interaction among pharmacists in large departments, and they are less isolated than in the past. Pharmacy colleges attempt to maintain tight control over preceptor programs to encourage students' clinical interests. Recent graduates of first pharmacy degree programs are encouraged to maintain contact with schools of pharmacy, even when employed, through the use of preceptorship programs where the newly licensed give on-the-job training to future pharmacists. As a result, linkages are maintained with the more idealistic and elite representatives of the field, those who advocate increased professionalization through the performance of clinical roles in health care. Opportunities for interaction help create an atmosphere of commitment to a cause, a strong sense of shared fate, and personal obligation to others who are similarly situated. These socially structured conditions promote the idea that pharmacy can and should undergo upgrading if it is to prevent loss of status and power.

Social Mobility Within Bureaucratized Health Care

Unlike medicine or engineering, pharmacy does not seek to become a dominant profession, merely to avoid dispossession. Yet the effort must be considered a collective mobility project "because only through a joint organizational effort could roles be created — or redefined — that would bring the desired social position to their occupants" (Larson 1977, 67).

Moreover, redefining the role of the pharmacist must occur within a highly complex health-care system. Given the structural changes discussed above, and the idiom by which status is expressed in the medically dominated health-care field in the United States, the direction this profession feels compelled to take is away from the technical and business components and toward the clinical service ideal.

The road that clinical pharmacy is taking, albeit rough, is not without precedent in health care. Redefinitions of technical functions as clinical services have occurred in the past. Anesthesiology, radiology and pathology, specialties once considered to be outside medicine, became defined as clinical services and increased their prestige (and incomes) by joining it. Pharmacy has no such goals at this time, but it is demanding more responsibility.

In fact, clinical pharmacy is something of a leader on the margins of the profession. Professional specializations in pharmacy do not represent interdependence in the same way that they do in medicine. Community pharmacists do not need to consult with hospital pharmacists. Each works in a different environment, with different opportunities for career advancement; and to some extent they are interchangeable operatives. Hospital pharmacists sometimes moonlight as chain-store pharmacists in order to earn additional income. Different because of their higher level of training, clinical pharmacists look to create support for their goals, within the field, as well as from physicians, hospital administrators, and third party payers.

To what extent are the physician assistants and nurse practitioners structurally similar to clinical pharmacists, and to what extent are they different? Pharmacy has the advantage of being able to set its own license requirements, without consulting the profession of medicine. In contrast, the other new professions in the shadow of medicine, called into being like sorcerers' apprentices, enjoy the protection of a sponsor; in this case, a sovereign profession. Clinical pharmacy must seek to find social approval and legitimation of its mission on its own. In a sense, it must win over the profession of medicine to its cause.

Physician associates face a different structural problem if they seek greater autonomy: They must demonstrate that they can deliver the services they were called on to deliver as well as their sponsors can; and to do an even better job, they must have more opportunity to "practice" in the community. Created by "corporate rationalizers" to end the shortage in primary-care providers in an age of (over) specialization, nurse practitioners, too seek that kind of opportunity, free of legal and financial restrictions. The next two chapters will deal with the search for autonomy for physician associates.

References

Adamcik, B. and others. 1986. "New clinical roles for pharmacists: A study of role expansion." *Social Science and Medicine* 23: 1187–1200.

Anonymous. 1973. "Communicating the value of comprehensive pharmaceutical services to the consumer." *Journal of the American Pharmaceutical Association* 23: NS13.

Anonymous. 1987. "Women flocking into pharmacy schools, graduate programs." *Drug Topics* 131 (August 3): 15–16.

Beckhard, R. 1972. "Organizational issues in the team delivery of comprehensive care." *Milbank Memorial Fund Quarterly* 50: (July) 287–316.

Begun, J.W., and R.D. Feldman. 1981. *A Social and Economic Analysis of Professional Regulation in Optometry.* Washington, D. C.:Center for Health Services Research.

Braverman, Harry. 1972. *Monopoly Capital and Labor.* New York: Monthly Review Press.

Broadhead, Robert S., and N.J. Facchinetti. 1985. "Drug iatrogenesis and clinical pharmacy: The mutual fate of a social problem and a professional movement." *Social Problems* 33: 425-436.

Cambridge Research Institute (CRI). 1975. *Trends Affecting the United States Health Care System.* Washington, D.C.: United States Government Printing Office.

Christansen, D.B., and P.J. Bush. 1981. "Drug Prescribing: Patterns, Problems and Proposals." *Social Science and Medicine* 15A: 343-355.

Cihlar, C. 1975. "Stephen L. Joyner, P.A." *Hospitals* 1 (June): 54.

Denzin, N. 1968. "Incomplete professionalization: The case of pharmacy." *Social Forces* 46: 375-381.

Glaser, M. 1987. "Exclusive new survey on pharmacists' salaries." *Drug Topics* 131 (October 5): 3-31.

Glazer, W. 1966. "Nursing leadership and policy." *The Nursing Profession: Five Sociological Essays,* edited by Fred Davis, 1-59. New York: Wiley.

Holcomb, B. 1988. "The druggists' crucial new role: Today's pharmacist must help people monitor their use of medication." *New York Times Good Health Magazine,* pt. 2 (April 17): 39-63.

Institute of Medicine. 1978. *A Manpower Policy for Primary Health Care.* Washington, D.C.: National Academy of Sciences.

Knapp, D.A. and D.E.Knapp. 1968. "An appraisal of the contemporary practice of pharmacy." *American Journal of Hospital Pharmacy* 32: 749.

Klegon, D. 1978. "The sociology of professions: An emerging perspective." *Sociology of Work and Occupations* 5: 259-283.

Kormel, B. 1978. "Hospital pharmacist: master or victim of the environment?" *American Journal of Hospital Pharmacy* 35: 151-154.

Kronus, C. 1975. "Occupational values, role orientation and work settings: The case of pharmacy." *Sociological Quarterly* 16: 171-183.

_____. 1976. "The evolution of occupational power: An historical study of task boundaries between physicians and pharmacists." *Sociology of Work and Occupations* 3: 3-37.

Lamy, P.O. 1978. "Pharmacy—today and tomorrow." *Contemporary Pharmacy Practice* 1: 1.

Larson, M. S. 1977. *The Rise of Professionalism: A Sociological Analysis.* Berkeley: University of California Press.

Light, D. W. 1986. "Surplus versus Containment: The changing context for health providers." In *Applications of Social Science to Clinical Medicine and Health Policy,* edited by Linda Aiken, and David Mechanic, 519-542. New Brunswick, N.J.: Rutgers University Press.

Love, D.W. and others. 1978. "Teaching interviewing skills to pharmacy residents." *American Journal of Hospital Pharmacy* 35: 1073-1074.

Lyons, R.C. 1979. "Incoming chief of drug agency." *New York Times* (September 12).

Mechanic, D. 1970. "Social issues in the study of the pharmaceutical field." *American Journal of Pharmacy Education* 34: 536-543.

Merton, R.K. 1958. "The functions of the professional association." *American Journal of Nursing* 58: 50-54.

National Associations of Boards of Pharmacy. 1987-1988. *Survey of Pharmacy Law Including all Fifty States, D.C., and Puerto Rico.* Park Ridge, Ill.: National Association of Boards of Pharmacy.

National Center for Health Statistics. 1985. *Health United States: 1985.* Washington, D.C.: Department of Health and Human Services.

Nelson, A.A., J.M. Meinhold, and R.A. Hutchinson. 1971. "Changes in physicians' attitudes toward pharmacists as drug information consultants following implementation of clinical pharmacy services." *American Journal of Hospital Pharmacy* 35: 1201-1206.

Provost, C. P. 1972. "Clinical pharmacy—specialty or general direction?" *Drug Intelligence and Clinical Pharmacy* 6: 235.

Rosenberg, Charles. 1987. *The Care of Strangers: The Rise of America's Hospital System.* New York: Basic Books.

Schneider, P. and G. Cable. 1978. "Compliance and clinical opportunity for an expanded practice role for pharmacists." *American Journal of Hospital Pharmacy* 35: 288-295.

Silver, George. 1976. *A Spy in the House of Medicine.* Germantown, Md.: Aspen Systems.

Smith, M. and D.A. Knapp. 1976. *Pharmacy, Drugs and Medical Care.* 2nd ed. Baltimore: Williams and Wilkins.

Starkweather, D.B. 1970. "Hospital size, complexity and formalization." *Health Services Research* 5 (Winter): 330-341.

Thompson, E.P. 1963. *The Making of the English Working Class.* New York: Vintage.

Zellmer, W.A. 1979. "Reviewing the 1970s: Hospital pharmacy practice." *American Journal of Hospital Pharmacy* 36: 1490.

Chapter 3

Reinventing Primary Care: The Training of Physician Extenders

As hospital care accounted for 39 percent of national health expenditures in 1974 (Cambridge Research Institute [CRI] 1975, 155), corporate rationalizers became increasingly concerned with ways to reduce the need for hospitalization. They reasoned that if an alternative form of care could be delivered on an outpatient basis, costs would be reduced. Thus, physician extenders were created by rising medical costs, to which the hospital system made a major contribution. But physician extenders provided new forms of care, and so a system had to be developed for their education and training. Different work settings soon emerged, as well as a distinct, although sometimes ambiguous, professional identity.

Planners also suggested that physicians might not have to evaluate and treat minor illness, educate and screen patients in order to prevent serious illness (e.g., hypertension), and monitor long-term posthospitalization recovery (Sadler, Sadler, and Bliss 1972, 10-11). Instead, under the supervision of physicians, nurse practitioners and physician assistants could handle some of the procedures, including physical examinations, acquiring detailed patient histories, performing diagnostic and therapeutic procedures, and even prescribing drugs under physicians' standing orders.

There are now 11,000 physician assistants and 15,000 nurse practitioners in the United States (Graduate Medical Education National Advisory Committee 1981). How were they recruited, and what were the outcomes of their training? Where did they come from? And does their experience resemble in any way the acquisition of knowledge, ability, and motivation by medical doctors?

Before I answer these questions, let me show how the increasing division of labor and new patterns of funding have pushed in the direction of still further specialization to compensate for gaps in services or expensive demands on the health-care system. Health care takes the second-largest share of the gross national product and is a major source of employment in the United States. More than 4 million people provide direct or indirect health-care services. The demand for health care seems endless, and the field of medicine encourages this expansion by taking on new tasks (e.g., the treatment of alcoholism), developing new technologies (e.g., body scanners), and identifying new diseases (e.g., hyperactivity in children). And if the 37 million Americans without health insurance receive some assistance from federal and state governments in the near future, the demand on the health-care system will be even greater than it is now. Physicians make up only 10 percent of the total number of health-care positions, and this proportion is expected to decline presently.

Traditionally, the physician was relieved of some work by delegating clerical and routine medical tasks to lesser-trained and lower-paid operatives. Dividing the complex from the simple meant that physicians could devote almost all of their time to using their most highly developed skills. Today the big cost saving is in avoiding hospitalization; we must rethink the conventional wisdom of using inpatient facilities for tasks that could be accomplished on an outpatient basis. In the 1990s there will be an increasing shift of labor in health care away from hospitals and into community practice settings. Now that the public has learned to trust hospitals, and health-care personnel are in place to run them, shifting services to outpatient care and the use of physician extenders is a daunting task. More than 70 percent of all health-care personnel work in general hospitals. For every hospital bed in these acute-care settings in the United States, there are 3.1 persons or full-time equivalents employed. ("Full-time equivalents" refer to half the hours worked by students or trainees, whose labor time is counted along with that of paid employees. See Silver 1976, 147). Labor costs account for 70 percent of the budget of major short-term general hospitals (Steton 1977, B18). In a paradoxical way, new technology in health care encourages employment rather than saving labor, since the standards of diagnosis and treatment are higher, meaning that more needs to be done.

The increase in the number of health-care employees has been matched by the proliferation of jobs in the field. More than 200 health care specialties are listed in the Department of Labor's *Dictionary of Occupational Titles.* In the late 1960s and early 1970s, articles in major medical journals advocated the creation of new health-care practitioners to help share the workload. The new technology not only resulted in many new positions, such as inhalation therapists and histologic or blood technicians, but these positions required assistants and aides. Occupational therapists, radiology technologists, and social workers were freed to do the more complicated work, while assistants took over routine assignments. As a joke in the 1970s said, even *Hamburger Helper* has an assistant!

These changes in the division of labor have occurred under the direction and control of physicians (CRI 1975, 328). Medicine itself has become increasingly specialized, with only 47 percent of all doctors now providing primary care. There are sixty-five AMA-approved medical specialties, and physicians in training seem to be avoiding primary care. In 1973, when the physician-extender movement was at its peak, only 37 percent of physicians in residency programs were in primary-care specialties (CRI 1975, 357). The creation of newer specialties, such as nurse practitioner and physician's assistant, resulted both from this shortage of primary care and from the control over the division of labor exercised by the profession of medicine.

Reimbursement at a flat rate and the development of prepaid insurance plans in the form of health maintenance organizations (HMOs) have encouraged the employment of physician extenders to do many of the tasks formerly done by doctors or house staff. The organization of care, when seen from the perspective of how tasks are divided and assigned, involves a delegation of responsibilities that once were exclusively those of physicians, mainly tasks performed by those in training (interns and residents). With fewer house staff, there is also less need for supervising or teaching physicians. The movement to diagnosis related groups (DRGs) only accelerated a movement that was already in place in the 1970s.

In order to keep costs down, or at least to give the appearance of being cost conscious, hospital management has had to innovate by replacing physicians with cheaper professionals.

Saward (1973) has suggested that the division of labor has been encouraged by the financing of health care, and will continue to produce new delegations of tasks from physicians to their surrogates.

> Present concepts of the role of the physician, the nurse and other health professionals will change rapidly under fixed budgeting for defined populations if different delivery systems are allowed to compete. If a technical tasks can be done by a nurse practitioner at a third of the cost of its being done by a physician, there will be an interest in the delegation of the task. (p.194)

Education and Training

By 1978, according to the Bureau of Health Manpower of the Department of Health and Human Services, there were fifty training programs for physician assistants (PAs), most of them aimed at primary care. That number has increased to fifty-four by 1987 (American Medical Association 1987). The physician assistant is trained to perform a variety of routine and delegated patient services under the supervision or direction of a physician. First established by Eugene A. Stead, M.D. at Duke University in 1966, the pilot training program lasted twenty-four months, with nine months of classroom instruction and fifteen months of clinical rotations (Wilson and Neuhauser 1985, 56).

The programs to train physician assistants then evolved into a three-year curriculum, involving a modified version of the first two years of medical school, with heavy emphasis on the basic sciences. Often, a general two-year junior college education is required before the study of anatomy, physiology, biochemistry, pharmacology, and related disciplines can begin. Clinic experiences are introduced during the second year and are expanded during the final year of internship in various ambulatory health services. At the end of the program, many academic-based students receive a baccalaureate degree. Three-year programs once took high school graduates, to train them to provide primary care without having the extensive knowledge of the medical doctor, thinking they would "have the educational background, clinical proficiency, competence and problem solving ability to make medical diagnoses, institute medical treatment and provide comprehensive preventive and primary therapeutic medical care and counseling" (Silver 1974, 97–98). Today, four-year baccalaureate programs are very common, replacing the "crash course" programs of the early days.

Increasingly, the PA was perceived as an inexpensive substitute for the trained medical professional. By 1977, Child Health Associates, a variant of the PA, were considered by observers to be fully prepared to diagnose competently and treat 90 percent of ambulatory pediatric patients five years after the completion of high school, at a cost of approximately one-fourth the expense of educating a pediatrician to perform the same tasks and functions (Ott and Knox 1977).

A nationwide survey of PA training programs was carried out in 1983 to determine the performance expected of students on graduation. Program directors were provided with a list of tasks reflecting primary-medical-care problems, and were asked to indicate what they expected their graduates to be able to do. With considerable congruence among directors, all students were expected to perform a patient history and physical examination, to establish a working diagnosis for the most common problems, and to formulate a management plan for many of them (Golden and Cawley 1983).

To become a nurse practitioner, a registered nurse must receive additional training, increasingly at the master's degree level. Training programs for nurse practitioners emphasize clinical and psychosocial counseling skills more than the basic sciences usually found in the curriculum for physician assistants. In 1975, forty-five academic programs awarded master's degrees to nurse practitioners. Today, 300 programs train nurse practitioners in the United States. Initially, programs that trained and certified nurse practitioners were almost exclusively located in hospitals; some registered nurses were trained and certified in tutorial programs worked out with physicians in solo or group practice. Crossover careers are possible for nurses and nurse practitioners; they are eligible to be certified as physician's assistants by passing a qualifying examination. Interestingly, the Office of Technology Assessment reported in 1986 that there were between 25,000 and 30,000 trained nurse practitioners in the United States, but only 15,500 were employed in their field of training (U.S. Office of Technology Assessment 1986). The demand for nurses in the United States continues to exceed the supply. Nurse practitioners often become managers or professors in nursing schools as a way of advancing their careers.

Henry Silver and his associates at the University of Colorado Medical School in 1968 began a training program for nurses who wished to become pediatric nurse practitioners (PNPs). Nurses who participated felt that their talents were more adequately utilized than they had been in the traditional nursing role. Using the curriculum model suggested by the University of Colorado group (Silver 1968, 298–302), Ruth Stein developed a program at Bronx Municipal Hospital Center in which registered nurses were given four months of lectures and demonstrations in pediatrics. This was followed by a twenty-month internship program for PNPs. During internship, trainees provided primary care under the supervision of a pediatrician and a certified nurse practitioner, with a progressive increase occurring in their patient panel and expanded responsibility and discretion in practice. This internship went beyond the academic training in Silver's model, where PNPs did not provide care for a panel of patients. The curriculum of the PNP training program was designed to prepare the former nurse for the major responsibility of providing primary comprehensive pediatric care. At the end of the program, the PNP was permitted to treat common minor illnesses; participate with physicians in the screening, evaluation, and management of more severe, acute, or chronic illnesses; and have multiple day-to-day contacts with various medical specialists in an acute-care hospital setting, thereby participating in carrying out treatment plans. In addition, PNPs were expected to develop an appreciation of the major psychosocial factors and the way they impinge on health-care delivery.

Recruitment to this special training program brought applicants whose major motivation was to overcome the compartmentalization of tasks found in modern hospital care and to "get more into" the clinical aspects of their roles as nurses. Becoming a PNP provided an opportunity for greater patient involvement, since the strategic focus of the role is the interface between patient, family, hospital, and various medical services. Later studies of recruits to nurse practitioner training programs found similar results. Hayden, Davies, and Clore (1982) found that respondents were motivated to enter an emergency nurse practitioner training program in order to gain greater role credibility, autonomy, and job advancement; to learn new skills; and to overcome strong dissatisfaction with present jobs.

In the original Bronx-based effort, all the nurses selected for the unit were experienced in handling a great deal of responsibility, such as working in a pediatric intensive care unit, supervising other nurses, or working in a hemodialysis program. The development of clinical responsibility as a PNP was different, however. Nurses at a particular station in a hospital had more organizational supports to rely on than other nurses, house staff, and PNPs providing primary care. A new sense of self was acquired by the PNPs; in 1974 a pediatrician who utilized a PNP in private practice said at a public forum that "nurses who have left for special training acquire a special aura about them; the nurse comes back a different person."

The Making of a Professional Identity

A new professional identity cannot be assigned; it has to emerge out of new responsibilities. Performing the role of PNP called into question the previous occupational identity of the nurse: (1) as the unquestioned subordinate to the physician; and (2) as the health-care agent whose day-to-day responsibilities are many but whose medical judgments and advice are not to be taken seriously. Accordingly, we would expect that a change in responsibilities would create a new professional identity. In one case study, patients cared more for nurse practitioners whose behavior "suggested an integration of medical and nursing care processes . . ." than for those who frequently sought physician consultation (Lewis and Cheyovich 1976, 365).

The participant observations reported in the following pages constitute a case study based on field work I conducted over a twelve-month period (Birenbaum 1974). Subjects in the study expressed their personal and professional concerns during the course of the working day, during team meetings, at several home visits when PNPs went to monitor patients and their families, and when physicians in other services had encounters with PNPs. Interviews also took place casually during the working day, and respondents usually expressed their own concerns rather than respond to issues expressly raised for their consideration, following the methods of Becker and Geer (1958).

The new sense of self acquired by PNPs parallels that of the medical students studied by Becker and his co-workers (1961, 234). Professional responsibility extended beyond being conscientious on duty; it included direct interaction with the client, with one's peers, and with other members of the team. Trainees learned how to use other members of the team, not just present cases to them. The objectives of the meeting were to develop treatment plans in the face of uncertain cooperation from other specialty units (e.g., Would the rehabilitation unit provide transportation for the family of a child with bilateral skull fractures?) The PNP learned to develop contingency plans since all the components of the initial plan were not guaranteed.

Once the plan was in place, the PNP became involved in executing treatments that were done under physicians' standing orders. When uncertain about treatment, PNPs consulted with the physicians in the program. All along the way, PNPs were required to explain to families what was going to happen next with respect to therapeutics or tests for the child. One of the great strengths of the program was the counseling and interpretation performed by PNPs.

Control over the dispensing of information to the client is a responsibility that often distinguishes the independent professional from others (Freidson 1970a, 141). PNPs were increasingly able to share this task with physicians; they explained the nature of the illness and the need for procedures to parents and child, and interpreted the results of diagnostic tests for them. It is important to note that not all physicians feel at ease when sharing their traditional rights and responsibilities. It can be said that physicians as well as physician extenders, have to learn to work in partnership. Some physicians have not developed the capacity to work with nontraditional providers in ways that would permit the fullest utilization of their skills and knowledge.

Perhaps of utmost significance was that the new responsibility brought a personal reorganization of the PNP's sense of identity: From a person who works on receiving orders to one who sets the pace of work and is self-directed; from a person who works toward a goal of getting a patient well to one who works toward a goal of keeping a patient well; from a person who sees work as giving advice as well as providing a service, and that the advice given is necessary for solving the patient's problem; and as a person whose job never ends, rather than one who can forget the job at the end of the day.

Thus, the PNPs acquired a different sense of work. As the scope of the role was extended, the direction of demands was reversed, and the demands themselves became far more reciprocal. PNPs not only made preliminary diagnoses but also set up the means by which these hypotheses could be confirmed, through laboratory tests or consultations with specialists. Continuous concern with the well-being of a child patient, beyond the initial bout of illness, was often demonstrated. Even after a child's medical problem was under control, PNPs took it upon themselves to followup on the child, to catch a reversal if one occurred.

Although PNPs established an ongoing relationship with the patient's family, they regarded themselves as providing a limited set of services. At first, families that did not follow a PNP's advice were often told that the PNP could "only go so far" if the family did not heed warnings about getting into counseling or changing family practices. But less experienced nurses were not able to set limits with families or withdraw support from a family that would not accept advice. Later, the physician in the program attempted to demonstrate that noncompliance could be based on factors outside the PNP's control. The development of a realistic perspective was helpful in getting PNPs not to regard every noncompliant parent as personally rejecting them, nor to feel that they were responsible for parents' negative behavior.

Still, PNPs, during the course of their training, began to feel that they were in charge of their patient panel. As one woman remarked, "This job is not just eight hours a day. I think about the cases all the time. I feel I am responsible for everything. It is really a mind-bending experience."

At the same time, the PNPs learned that immediate and constant availability to patients is not a demonstration of responsibility. Initially, staff meetings were interrupted by phone calls and messages from secretaries, saying that a patient's mother wanted to speak to a PNP or had shown up without an appointment and was waiting outside. Staff M.D.s stressed that being well prepared is more important than giving immediate attention, unless it is an emergency; that responsibility as a concept extends beyond one's patients and to the staff as well; that PNPs should have some control over scheduling; and that self-mastery is an important aspect of being an independent professional. PNPs began to learn that *when* to act and *how* to act were matters of acquiring judgment.

Independent Judgment

One of the central features of an independent professional is the capacity to use judgment in situations that are not clear-cut or in cases where the extension of one's service and advice may be problematic. The appearance of a client with a problem is not always a direct signal that intervention is possible. A large part of the training of an independent professional is learning when and where to attempt "solutions to the concrete problems of individuals" (Freidson 1970b, 163).

One aspect of the PNP's training was to learn how to recognize limitations. The medical practitioner must be able to tell when a difficult case requires an experienced or specialized physician. The practitioner should regard this as a sign of competency, not incompetency; one must know when one's poor judgment might endanger the patient. The physician himself is frequently faced with a similar decision in referrals to specialists. And no one questions the competence of a physician who uses specialized consultants.

Self-limitation, as an aspect of judgment, became part of an orientation to work. The PNPs understood that some patients will not respond to their services. They had to demonstrate that their right to accept or reject a case was respected by the medical staff of the training program (Freidson 1970a, 121). In providing home care for a chronically ill child, for example, the PNP had to make sure that the parents would provide day-to-day care. Sometimes the PNP might feel that the child was better off in the hospital, as in the following observations:

> The staff meeting centered around discussion of cases not to be included in the program. In one case, the mother was inconsistent in taking the child's pulse and in giving digitalis. An aunt of the child was to be trained to do this, but when she was visiting the child on the ward with the mother, she did nothing but act as a translator. A PNP said that she "was a long way away from picking up this child" and no one questioned her judgment.

Sometimes the service would take a child on a trial basis, provided that additional services could be arranged. In the area of planning, the PNP's judgment was respected by physicians. When a physician presented the details of a prospective case, the PNP made contributions and suggested procedures to use when in contact with the patient. In contrast, during the early part of training, PNPs were often unsure of how involved they should get with families, would never offer suggestions to doctors, or would withdraw services from uncooperative families.

The training program, both in the formal curriculum and the behaviors it encouraged, imparted a new way of working with medical practitioners and patients. These empowering experiences have influenced efforts on the part of nurse practitioners to seek to expand their role in the direction of greater autonomy, a topic discussed in chapter 4. It is highly unlikely that nurse practitioners will ever become completely independent of the discipline of medicine. Some autonomy may be acquired, to the extent that the PNP achieves the right to engage in a limited community practice. But it is not likely that, as a profession, the nurse practitioner will achieve a "legal monopoly over performance of some strategic aspect of work and effectively prevents free competition from other occupations" (Freidson 1970a, 123). Nevertheless, it is possible, if not easy to convince related professionals, that nurse practitioners can best perform the services they provide and should have a legal monopoly over that performance.

There is evidence that the new roles are regarded by the performers as involving activities far removed from traditional nursing. A quantitative study of the expanded role of the nurse practitioner (NP) found that the NP more frequently performed functions previously unknown to the nursing profession, such as physical assessment and prescription of medications (Vacek and Ashikaga 1980).

Whether the training occurred in a hospital-based program or through a nursing school master's program seemed to make little difference on employment patterns among nurse practitioners. Work-related activities and professional tasks in one study were similar for PNP-employed graduates, regardless of educational level. Nonmaster's-prepared NPs were more likely to be employed in primary health-care delivery settings and live in rural locations (Cruikshank and Lakin 1986). Education may serve as a self-selection factor, as far as work and living location are concerned, rather than be used by employers to differentiate according to skill level.

The role content, however, has been found to be affected by differences in education. In another study comparing master's and nonmaster's prepared PNPs, the study authors found that the better educated were more likely to do assessments of physical and cognitive development of infants, assessments of personality and socialization of preschool children, and counseling and guidance involving the physical and cognitive development of infants. Professional activity also seems to be related to level of education. The better educated PNPs were more likely than the nonmaster's PNPs to be engaged in leadership activities within the profession of nursing (Glascock, Webster-Stratton, and McCarthy 1985).

A sense of having new responsibilities has consistently been found to be a source of stress to new nurse practitioners. The broad definition of the role often leaves the occupant uncertain as to what he or she should implement in practice and what remains the province of the doctor (Rapson 1982). In a survey of 135 NPs, adjustment to new responsibilities was indicated as taking approximately six months. Respondents felt that uncertainty about the diagnosis and treatment of patients and fear of overlooking disease when it was present were the most distressing feelings experienced (Lukacs 1982). These emotions are not unlike those experienced by medical students and interns. Doctors, in their training, learn to identify disease and err on the side of seeing it present when it is *not* there, rather than overlooking symptoms when they are present.

Evaluation of Performance

Two major concerns about physician extenders have been (1) whether nurse practitioners and physician assistants would remain within the defined limits of their roles or would seek to expand them into new areas; and (2) whether they would perform as well as physicians in identifying and managing illness. The physicians who began training programs wanted to not only prove that their trainees were talented but also to reassure their colleagues that the new practitioners would not threaten their authority (or income).

In 1968, when Henry Silver and his associates at the University of Colorado Medical School began a training program for nurses who wished to become pediatric nurse practitioners, participants felt that their talents were more adequately utilized than they had been in the traditional nursing role. Nevertheless, trainees were careful to note that the boundary between what they did and what physicians did was still carefully drawn: "The limits of our activities are clearly defined. We do not pretend to function beyond these boundaries" (Stearly and others 1967, 2087). It would seem that today, nurse practitioners no longer think this way.

By 1980, the humble statement above no longer represented the spirit of the nurse practitioner movement. Rapid growth had occurred in a single decade, with 15,000 NPs in practice by 1979 and a projection of 31,000 by 1990 (Graduate Medical Education National Advisory Committee 1981). Moreover, the challenges to what has been the traditional "turf" of medicine have been undertaken by NPs in numerous instances, with some court decisions (e.g., *Sermchief* v. *Gonzales*, Missouri, 1984) supporting the concept that the tasks that nurses were performing (e.g., Pap smears) were within the confines of nursing, not just medicine. Moreover, the court ruled in *Sermchief* v. *Gonzales* that nurses had the right to diagnose and to administer medications prescribed by a licensed person (Schwartz, deWolf, and Skipper 1987, 566).

Of considerable importance in the politics of this movement has been the adoption of nurse practitioners by the profession of nursing. At one time NPs, were seen as rebels and deserters from nursing, but now they are cast into leadership roles and are models for the entire profession. Instead of being elite dropouts, NPs are considered to be carving out the future for nursing. The AMA's task force on physician extenders has been very careful to separate their findings and recommendations on PAs from their report on NPs because of the complicated boundary issues raised by one profession telling another profession what it can or cannot do.

Roles expansion will inevitably involve conflict if it is perceived as threatening to another profession's traditional tasks and prerogatives. A physician-extenders role, by definition, is meant to replace a traditional practitioner. One reason why role expansion took place is that evaluations of the skills of NPs, right from the start, were based on comparisons with the skills of medical doctors. The University of Colorado Medical School group compared the diagnoses of PNPs with those of physicians in 278 instances (Duncan and others 1971, 1170–1176). In only two cases were differences in judgment considered serious enough to affect the child's health status.

Similarly, physician assistant skills were subject to evaluation. In the Kaiser-Permanente plan on the West Coast, PAs are employed as primary-care providers. In one of these HMOs, a study of 207 patient-physician assistant encounters concluded with the PA taking care of patient needs for 166 cases without physician consultation. Discussion was required in 17 cases and referral to a physician in 24 instances (Lairson and others, 1974, 215).

These early findings are only the beginning of a movement to establish cognitive credibility for the burgeoning physician-extender field. Reception by the medical profession of the new practitioners has been mixed, however. In some instances, the work of physician extenders has been used to justify limiting surgical residencies in hospitals, since currently there is clearly an oversupply of trained surgeons in the United States. Physician assistants are now being trained to replace interns and residents in teaching hospitals that have cut back on the training of surgeons (Sullivan 1980). This effort is part of a national campaign of the American College of Surgeons to reduce competition in their field. This accrediting body also claims that nonsurgically trained physicians should not be permitted to have operating room privileges in hospitals because they are not sufficiently skilled, and do not have the opportunity to perform surgical procedures frequently enough to retain existing skills (Snoke 1987).

More frequently, we find instances where physician extenders are seen as pushing the boundaries of medicine when they perform primary-care functions. This conflict is not limited to the physician extender-physician relationship. Boundary disputes occur all the time between medical and nonmedical practitioners who perform similar functions or who make claims to heal using unorthodox (e.g., chiropractic) techniques. Physicians often jealously guard their exclusive rights to diagnose and treat disease. Opthamologists have opposed legislation that would permit optometrists to use drugs in order to diagnose eye disease: "Optometrists currently are not adequately or properly trained in the diagnosis of eye disease. Those in practice have had very limited exposure (if any exposure) to qualified training in the recognition of disease processes" (Taffet 1976, 27). Recently, psychiatrists have been resisting the inroads of clinically trained psychologists who seek affiliations with psychoanalytic institutes or wish to have admitting privileges in acute-care and specialty hospitals (Goleman 1988, B6). Freud, the founder of psychoanalysis and a physician himself, never sought to make this technique the exclusive tool of medicine. He fought, even with his disciples, to permit trained lay analysts to practice (Gay 1988). He might have thought differently today with all the competition in the field of psychoanalysis, just as the creators of physician extenders, the professional medical associations, are reconsidering their position on independence in practice for their creations.

Second Thoughts: the AMA Reviews Control

In 1969, during the time when the physician shortage was first seen by health-care planners as a serious problem, the AMA endorsed innovation and experimentation in developing new roles in health care. By 1979, in the midst of the physician glut, the AMA special task force set up to review developments in the area of physician and allied health manpower was dubious about the need for any further growth in the numbers of physician assistants and nurse practitioners in the United States. In fact, it recommended that public funding for programs to train physician assistants be opposed by the AMA. Furthermore, although the AMA endorsed the concept of "negotiated autonomy," the emphasis was more on the physician's right to remain free of legislative delineation of specific tasks that the PA could or could not do, rather than on the recognized skills of the physician extender (Anonymous 1981, 313).

Utilization of the PA was to be made subject to the approval of the state medical licensing board, to which a plan had to be submitted, detailing the proposed use of the PA, the qualifications of both the supervising physician and the PA, and a description of the practice setting. The task force recommended that supervision be direct, involving the personal presence of the physician, except in unusual practice settings where a state medical board waiver could be granted on a case-by-case basis. This position on the direct supervision and personal presence or participation by the physician in all instances where the physician extender provides services is a reversal from the AMA's early position that the personal presence of the physician was not necessary for adequate supervision (Anonymous 1981, 314). Organized medicine appears to be trying to control the runaway doctors in the profession as much as the new practitioners.

On the subject of whether PAs should be allowed to prescribe drugs, the task force recommended "opposition to legislation or proposed regulations authorizing physician's assistants to make independent medical judgments as to the drug of choice for an individual patient" (p.316). Prescribing can still occur "under standing orders."

Control over the dispensing of health care in the United States could be in the hands of a sovereign profession, or the related institutions could employ professionals and their surrogates. By employing PAs, hospitals could offer services that would cut into the market for health services now ruled by physicians. The task force was as concerned about the autonomy of medicine as it was about the PA's negotiated autonomy. The physician extender could serve patients of the supervising physician in all types of health-care settings (e.g., nursing homes, patient's homes), but the state medical board would determine just how many PAs a single doctor could employ. Concern was expressed that hospitals employing PAs directly could not always provide good medical supervision. With 27 percent of the graduates of AMA-approved programs finding employment in hospitals, the task force was also concerned about the varied tasks and supervisory conditions under which PAs worked: "For PAs exercising independent judgment, the Task Force believes that direct supervision by a designated responsible physician rather than by a health care institution is critical to optimum patient care" (Anonymous 1981, 315). The task force took no position on *who* should be the employer, the doctor or the hospital, but realized that this was something that required an AMA policy statement.

Nurse practitioners have not been subject to new policy statements that limit their autonomy in practice, but progress has not been spectacular for these physician extenders. Independent prescribing has moved slowly for nurse practitioners, despite their enthusiasm for modification of state prescription laws. There have even been some major setbacks for the NPs; one such recently occurred in California when the legislature defeated a move to liberalize prescription laws and regulations. Since 1975, however, eighteen states have modified their laws to permit limited but independent prescription authority to be wielded by NPs (Manber 1985). The AMA has spoken out to prevent changes in legislation that would permit nonmedical providers to perform medical tasks.

There are many policy questions about the utilization of non-physicians that are still unanswered. A major conference on the subject, sponsored by the National Center for Health Services Research and the Bureau of Health Manpower, concluded that communications studies are required to "further understand the nature of the communication process and the patient and provider variables which interact with this process to produce specific health outcomes" (U.S Department of Health and Human Services 1979, 12). This is not only an important subject for review, and in the next chapter I examine the ways in which physician extenders have sought to make good their claims that the work they do is not only important, but of as good or better quality, than the work of medical doctors.

References

American Medical Association (AMA). 1987. *Allied Health Directory.* 15th ed. Chicago: American Medical Association.

Anonymous. 1981. "AMA policy on physician's assistants." *Connecticut Medicine* 45 (May): 311–317.

Becker, Howard, and others.1961. *Boys in White: Student Culture in Medical School.* Chicago: University of Chicago Press.

Becker, H., and B. Geer. 1958. "Problems of inference and proof in participant observation." *American Sociological Review* 23 (December): 652–60.

Birenbaum, A. 1974. "The making of a professional identity: The pediatric nurse practitioner." *Sociological Symposium* 11 (Spring): 98–118.

Cambridge Research Institute (CRI). 1975. *Trends Affecting the U.S. Health Care System.* Washington, D.C.: Department of Health, Education, and Welfare.

Cruikshank, B.M., and J.A. Lakin. 1986. "Professional and employment characteristics of NPs with master's and non- master's preparation." *Nursing Practice* 11 (November): 45–52.

Duncan, B., and others. 1971. "Comparison of the physical assessment of children by pediatric nurse practitioners and pediatricians." *American Journal of Public Health* 61 (June): 1170–1176.

Freidson, Eliot. 1970a. *Professional Dominance: The Social Structure of Medical Care.* New York: Atherton Press.

_____. 1970b. *The Profession of Medicine: A Study of the Sociology of Applied Knowledge.* New York: Dodd, Mead.

Gay, Peter. 1988. *Freud: A Life for Our Time.* New York: Norton.

Glascock, J.C., C. Webster-Stratton, and A.M. McCarthy. 1985. "Infant and preschool well-child care: Master's and nonmaster's prepared pediatric nurse practitioners." *Nursing Research* 34 (January/February): 39–43.

Golden, A.S., and J.F. Cawley. 1983. "A national survey of performance objectives of physician's assistant training programs." *Journal of Medical Education* 58 (May): 418–424.

Goleman, D. 1988. "Psychologists and psychiatrists clash over hospital and training barriers." *New York Times* (May 17): B6.

Graduate Medical Education National Advisory Committee. 1981. *Report of the Graduate Medical Education National Advisory Committee to the Secretary, Department of Health and Human Services.* Washington, D.C.: AAMC.

Hayden, M.L., L.R. Davies, and E.R. Clore. 1982. "Facilitators and inhibitors of the emergency nurse practitioner role." *Nursing Research* 31 (September/October): 294–299.

Lairson, P., J. Record, and J. James. 1974. "Physician assistants at Kaiser: Distinctive patterns of practice." *Inquiry* (September): 207–219.

Lewis, C.E. and T.K. Cheyovich. 1976. "Who is a nurse practitioner? Processes of care and patients' and physicians' perceptions." *Medical Care* 14: 365–371.

Lukacs, J.L. 1982. "Factors in nurse practitioner role adjustment." *Nursing Research* 7 (March): 21–23.

Manber, M.M. 1985. "NPs, MDs and PAs: Meshing their changing roles." *Medical World News* 26 (September 23): 53–71.

Ott, J.E., and G.K. Knox. 1977. "Costs of educating child health associates." *Annual Conference on Research on Medical Education* 16: 251–255.

Rapson, M.F. 1982. "Role stress of nurse practitioners." *Nursing Practice* 7 (July/August): 48–50.

Sadler, A.M., B.L. Sadler, and A.A. Bliss. 1972. *The Physician's Assistant: Today and Tomorrow.* New Haven: Yale University Press.

Saward, E.W. 1973. "Organization of medical care." *Scientific American* (September): 169–75.

Schwartz, H.D., P.L. deWolf, and J.K. Skipper. 1987. "Gender, professionalization, and occupational anomie: The case of nursing." In *Dominant Issues in Medical Sociology,* edited by Howard D. Schwartz, 559–569. 2nd. ed. New York: Random House.

Silver, George. 1976. *A Spy in the House of Medicine.* Germantown, Md.: Aspen Systems.

Silver, H.K. 1974. "New health professionals for primary ambulatory care." *Hospital Practice* (April): 97–98.

Silver, H.K., L.C. Ford, and L.R. Day. 1968. "The pediatric nurse practitioner program: Expanding the role of the nurse to private increased health care for children." *Journal of the American Medical Association* 204 (April): 298–302.

Snoke, Albert W. 1987. *Hospitals, Health and People.* New Haven: Yale University Press.

Stearly, S., A. Noordenbus, and V. Crouch. 1967. "Pediatric nurse practitioner." *American Journal of Nursing* 67 (October): 2083–2087.

Steton, D. 1977. "Hospital workers win pay increase." *New York Times* (June 29): B18.

Sullivan, R. 1980. "Help for the harried hospital doctors." *New York Times* (March 22): 23, 25.

Taffet, S. 1976. "Forum: For better eye care." *Mamaroneck Daily Times* (February 16): 27.

U.S. Department of Health and Human Services. 1979. *Nurse Practitioners and Physician Assistants: A Research Agenda.* Publication 79-3236. Washington, D.C.: Department of Health and Human Services.

U.S. Office of Technology Assessment. 1986. *Nurse Practitioners, Physician Assistants and Certified Nurse-Midwives: A Policy Analysis.* Technology Case Study 37. Washington, D.C.: Government Printing Office.

Vacek, P., and T. Ashikaga. 1980. "Quantification of the expanded role of the nurse practitioner: a discriminant analysis approach." *Health Services Research* 15 (Summer): 105–125.

Wilson, Florence, and Duncan Neuhauser. 1985. *Health Services in the United States.* Cambridge, Mass.: Ballinger.

4 **Social Approval of Physician Extenders and Institutional Barriers**

The major social trends in American society toward greater access to basic kinds of services, such as minimum support for children and the elderly, were framed in the social policies of the New Deal. Since World War II, the gains of people employed by others, not just the destitute, have extended to benefits collectively bargained for that have gone beyond maintaining the purchasing power of professional, technical, managerial, or blue-collar workers. For the poor, the gains have come from a recognition that health is a social, not a medical, concept. Failure to provide care for the needy means that those who are independent may be threatened by communicable diseases or epidemics. In addition, when health-care institutions such as hospitals provide uncompensated care, they may go so deeply in debt that they will not remain viable systems for dispensing services to all who need them, even paying clients. For all these reasons, health care has become viewed as a right of citizenship and not just a privilege; it is also seen as a necessity in a complex, interdependent society; and it becomes part of the public-sector's responsibilities to finance service delivery.

Along with ending the limited access to physicians by Americans who were poor or near-poor came a need to expand the labor force of the health-care system. No longer is health care seen as the exclusive province of medicine. More significantly, the creation of physician-extender roles has called into question whether independent judgment in health decisions should reside only with the highly trained physician. When nurse practitioners or physician assistants work in remote rural areas or urban ghettoes where there are few physicians, independent judgment is a necessity.

76

Relationships between doctors and physician extenders take a variety of forms. A fruitful collaboration between the new practitioner and the doctor need not be based on direct supervision as long as enough time is set aside for consultation and evaluation of performance. In fact, physical separation is made possible, if not actually encouraged, by state laws. In some states, the physician assistant and nurse practitioner can legally make house calls, prescribe medication for minor illnesses, and perform physical examinations. As a result, criteria for training have also been established in many states, perhaps before all the evidence is available on what the new practitioners can and cannot do well.

That physician assistants and nurse practitioners have some autonomy does not imply that all new health-care roles will be structured with similar independence. The conditions that allow independent judgment by these practitioners do not apply to other paramedical personnel who work under the physician's supervision. The new role of medical assistant, for example, has been created in order to relieve doctors of routine office tasks, such as measuring blood pressure, establishing height and weight, and taking blood samples (Fowler 1977). It may not be long before the physician's office will be similar to that of the dentist's, where the dental hygienist performs many paramedical duties.

Physician-extender roles were designed by corporate rationalizers to increase the doctor's reach, either by having a routine procedure delegated or by simple augmentation of the basic clinical services available. Critical to the success of this innovation is widespread acceptance by the medical world, leading to employment in various settings and patient use of the new practitioners. This chapter first reviews physician acceptance of the PA and NP, the formation of working relationships, and new forms of utilization. Next, patient approval is examined. Finally, the barriers to wider use of nurse practitioners are reviewed in the context of licensing restrictions and third-party reimbursement. Some insights are provided into the response of professional associations to role expansion.

It is my thesis that the physician-extender innovation, unlike clinical pharmacy, was widely accepted by physicians and patients long before all the evidence was in that the skills were there to perform the tasks assigned. Yet this was almost predictable given that medicine, with its cultural authority, called the physician extenders into being. The legitimacy of the innovator — the profession of medicine — overrode much of the public's skepticism. Control over the division of labor in health care appeared to be the special property of medicine, almost like a natural right, rather than historically derived. Furthermore, the legitimators engaged in the validation of the experiment, since physicians often served as research investigators, making comparisons of the skills of PAs and NPs with their peers. Most important, approval was forthcoming because performers were able to maintain favorable impressions, despite presenting a potential economic threat to the welfare of physicians by replacing them as providers of primary care.

In contrast, clinical pharmacists, by virtue of their narrow construction of the role, receive very little physician approval, even though they are not an economic threat to physicians. The rank of medicine is without peer in the world of health care, and it can confer or deny whatever status it wishes to its subordinates. In essence, clinical pharmacists may be first-rate professionals stuck in a second-tier profession. In contrast, the PA and NP were sponsored by medicine. The nurse practitioner movement has since moved closer to nursing; but as I later show, not all advances for the NP are applauded by the organized profession of nursing. The structural opportunities for a collective mobility project among PAs is limited by their being controlled by the profession of medicine.

The first kind of autonomy among NPs and PAs was the granting of what is called "institutional licensing," permitting the extender to diagnose and treat patients as outpatients or inpatients under standing orders. By 1990 some states certified nurse practitioners, allowing them to write prescriptions. Certification was based on pharmacology education, supervised clinical experience, and an ongoing practice agreement with a collaborating physician. Not working under direct supervision, the PA and NP in a hospital, nursing home, or clinic can see patients and carry a caseload, even when the doctor who wrote the orders is not on the premises. Admiration for the work of physician extenders was forthcoming in these very special and limited arrangements.

Physician Approval

Whether physicians are in favor or opposed to physician extenders, there is widespread agreement among them that their approval is a prerequisite to the extender's capacity to function effectively (Claiborn and Walton 1979, 300). Since physicians have traditionally been willing to delegate routine tasks, many leaders of organizational medicine were early advocates of these roles (Vox Paed 1978). The AMA has been the lead organization in developing accreditation for physician-assistant training programs. The expanded role of a nurse practitioner is also viewed by the Graduate Education Medical National Advisory Committee (GEMNAC) as one that provides direct patient care, involving independent decision making and collaboration with physicians and other providers (U.S. Office of Technology Assessment 1986, 12).

The basis for approval by the early advocates took two forms. First, with regard to the PA, medical providers emphasized increasing practice productivity while reducing the costs of service delivery. Second, the NP was perceived as being able to improve the quality of care through more intensive psychosocial training and a willingness to deal with patients on a day-to-day basis. The latter argument was a not-so-subtle criticism of the detachment from caring that some observers of medical services noted among physicians (Light 1986, 525). The result was that approval of these somewhat different providers by the medical profession was based on contradictory grounds. Efficiency could be gained by the delegation of routine tasks; effectiveness could be achieved by hiring a practitioner who was willing and able to get to know the patient and his or her family. As mentioned earlier, the AMA gave its strong endorsement to the creation of the PA and did not oppose the expanded nursing role of the NP.

Relationships between Physician Extenders and Physicians

When nurses first saw the opportunity to become nurse practitioners, nurses who wanted increasing intellectual responsibility and more recognition for the work they did responded positively. A question remained whether their relationship with doctors would continue to be one of subordination, dependence, and exclusion from decision making. The experience of working closely with doctors has helped dispel the notion that it is impossible to share responsibility and decision making. This conclusion does not mean that all doctors can work with nurse practitioners. The new collaboration is a good example of social selection. Physicians who opposed the development of physician-extender roles eschew contact with the "enemy," thereby making the experiences of these new physician extenders very satisfactory. In addition, being predisposed to hire a PA or NP makes a physician's attitude favorable to the physician-extender concept (Burkett and others 1978).

Previous experience in working with a physician extender predisposes physicians to hire them and be willing to delegate tasks to them (Lawrence and Others 1977). In a statewide study, 68 percent of North Carolina doctors who had previously worked with a nurse practitioner were more willing to hire one than the average of 34 percent of all doctors in the study. In addition, those with previous experience of working with NPs had higher task-delegation scores. A national probability sample of physicians surveyed by mail in the late 1970s found a strong demand for PAs, despite the limited numbers of graduates available for employment (Scheffler and Gillings 1982).

There is some evidence to suggest that the NP has an advantage over the PA. In a study of HMO physicians serving 270,000 subscribers, the preference for NPs was higher than that for PAs. Johnson and Freeborn (1986) found that "physicians felt that nurse practitioners were more likely to increase the quality of care and less likely to increase the risk of malpractice"(p.39). While this is only one study, its results suggest that physicians view the NP as a more adequate substitute for themselves in primary care.

The reality of physician–nurse practitioner contacts was more variable than one would suppose. In a follow-up study of graduates from a single program in California, Little (1980) found a range of relationships between physicians and NPs, from collegiality to treating the physician extender as a "guest" in the medical practice. Young physicians who were patient (not disease) oriented allowed NPs the greatest autonomy. Under these conditions, the NPs did not consider themselves nurses but peers with the physicians, limited only by licensing and legal requirements. In other relationships, NPs were far less in control of their patients, restricted by either bureaucratic or personal forms of control over the work that they were allowed to perform.

Physician acceptance varies somewhat when NPs and PAs are compared. Aside from the enormous difference that personal contact makes, the NP is perceived by physicians as capable of less than the nurse has been trained to do. To some extent, this may reflect physician caution in allowing NPs to do many things. The new physician-extender roles are responded to with some professional ambivalence by doctors. In private practice, they may approve an NP's performance in history taking or some other relatively simple task, but draw the line at the more difficult clinical judgment-based problem solving (U.S. Office of Technology Assessment 1986, 21). NPs who work in the more cost-conscious HMOs are permitted to do far more than simply take patient histories.

Actual descriptions of physicians' attitudes toward physician extenders reinforce the hierarchy of health care. To some in medicine, the NP is seen as a threat to the physician's relationships with patients. And the nurse's quest for autonomy is responded to negatively because it is perceived largely to be at the doctor's expense.

Less of a threat to the authority of medicine and its income-generating capacities are the physician assistants. Again, physicians trust the extenders once they get to know them and are willing to permit PAs to treat the patient who comes in unexpectedly to the office with an urgent problem when the physician is unavailable. Physicians also perceive the PA having greater skills than the NP precisely in those areas where NPs take great pride: Patient education, counseling, or instruction (U.S. Office of Technology Assessment 1986, 23).

Despite the limited acceptance given to NPs, observers of the relationship who write both as participants and as researchers in nursing journals describe the relationship as collegial (Choi 1981; Little 1980) or as a model of collaboration in pediatric care (Pierce, Quattlebaum, and Corley 1985). Brown (1979) observed that "one of the most satisfying trends I've seen is the development of working relationships between nurse practitioners and new resident doctors" (p. 78).

To what extent is a new division of labor emerging in primary care? Levine and others (1976) reported that in a prepaid group, new health practitioners (physician extenders) delivered over 75 percent of the well-person care, 56 percent of the problem-oriented care in adult medicine, and 29 percent of the problem-oriented children's care. In addition, they observed that physician extenders became increasingly involved in acute care, while physicians retained their dominant role in treating serious chronic illnesses.

The division of labor involves the conduct of communication as well as the distribution of tasks (Kane 1976). Other studies have focused on the extent to which interaction was dominated by physicians. Lamb and Napodano (1984) measured team interaction patterns between NPs and doctors in primary-care practices. They found little interaction between practitioners and minimal physician initiation of exchange on the team. Lewis and Cheyovich (1976) found that NPs who were more aggressive in interaction with patients were more likely to be perceived by patients and physicians as performing a new and innovative role.

New Forms of Utilization

One of the most striking expressions of physician approval of NPs and PAs is the development of variants from the basic theme of physician extender. One use of physician extenders that has been advocated is as a way of reducing the number of residents providing high-quality care in teaching hospitals and later going out and establishing specialty practices in overcrowded fields (Silver and McAtee 1984, 326). Surgical assistants (SAs) are trained PAs who learn surgical subjects in special programs. Approximately one-third of all PAs are now employed in this capacity (Greenberg 1984). As mentioned earlier, SAs now permit hospitals to end internship and residency programs in surgery, a specialty with an oversupply of practitioners.

Every innovation of this kind is a double-edged sword in medicine and surgery. The new hand that heals also is perceived as a threat to the existing profession. In replacing house staff, SAs are watched very carefully by the American College of Surgeons, to keep them from performing surgery and supervising junior medical doctor residents in surgery. In this highly crowded specialty, the American College of Surgeons is equally aware that physicians who assist in operating rooms are now competing with surgeons, and they fear that SAs may soon be doing the same thing (Hanlon 1980, 243).

Another clinical innovation involves NPs in a special training program to learn how to assume the care of patients undergoing cardiopulmonary bypass surgery. Now designated physician's clinical associates (PCAs), nurse practitioners with extensive experience in critical care become "responsible for the detailed management of all cardiac surgical patients from admission to discharge, except during the first 48 hours postoperatively when they are managed by staff physicians in the intensive care unit" (Weiland 1983, 578). PCAs do much of the preparatory work for the cardiac unit on the admission or transfer of a patient, including writing preoperative orders, taking complete medical histories, physical examinations, reviewing laboratory data, and ordering any indicated vascular studies. In addition, PCAs give information to patients and their families, do preliminary diagnosis, and provide psychosocial support when needed. Following surgery, PCAs, with physician consultation, manage clear-cut problems such as urinary tract infection, pulmonary congestion, or insulin readjustment for chronic diabetes (Weiland 1983, 578).

Perhaps no specialty in medicine has been more sympathetic to the NP than pediatrics has been to the pediatric nurse practitioner (PNP). Recommendations of the American Academy of Pediatrics (AAP) speak to the need for PNPs and their important contribution to child health care (Vox Paed 1978, 740). Joint statements of the AAP and the American Nursing Association (ANA) call the relationship between pediatrician and PNP a model of collaboration between medicine and nursing. Here it is clear that the PNP is not replacing the heavily burdened pediatricians, only extending care to underserved populations.

Similarly, the demand for neonatal intensive care services, combined with an undersupply of trained neonatologists, has lead to a willingness to train PNPs in Level III neonatology, which deals with infants at highest risk (Robertson 1983, 264).

Creating Credibility

Sponsored professions have a distinct advantage over newly developed professions, such as clinical pharmacy, since the high-status profession can delegate whatever it wishes. Since medicine controlled the birth of both the NP and the PA, it determined whether the quality of services delivered by physician extenders was as good as that provided in primary care by experienced physicians. The new health-care providers were subject to evaluation research, designed, for example, to determine (1) whether the NP or PA was as careful or as thorough as a physician (process measures) or (2) had the same impact on patient (compliance with treatment regimens) and health outcome measures.

In seeking to determine outcomes, measures are taken on populations that have received a new service that is being evaluated and compared to populations where traditional ways of doings things obtain. Outcome measures and controls are extremely difficult to establish and take a lot of time to perfect; nevertheless, they provide hard evidence that something works. To document that designated consequences follow from the work of physician extenders, an outcome study may be employed to compare their work with that of physicians. Controls are not likely to be built into such a design, as they might be in clinical drug trials, but some effort is made to limit random effects. Unlike theoretically relevant research, outcome studies do not try to explain how and why something works; they answer only the pragmatic question of *whether* it works.

The process measure does not deal with the question of end results, but of whether the service was delivered in a professionally appropriate way. For example, are PAs able to follow a protocol correctly? Do NPs prescribe correctly for diagnosed minor illnesses? Both outcome and process measures serve as a form of quality assurance that goes beyond determining that NPs or PAs received the appropriate training and education.

The reinvention of primary care has called for the creation of numerous studies of the skills and impacts of the physician extenders. As can be seen in Tables 4.1 and 4.2, both process and outcome studies have been conducted for well over fifteen years. There are many weaknesses in the published studies, mainly because they used small samples, depended on short-term outcomes, used nonrandomized study populations, and applied single-evaluation criteria (U.S. Office of Technology Assessment 1986, 18). In addition, the comparison group of doctors in some of the studies was limited to hospital house staff, rather than seasoned physicians. Still, these studies provide evidence that the quality of care by NPs and PAs, within the limits of their training, is as good as that provided by physicians. In two important areas, resolving patients' acute problems and prescribing, NPs were found to do just as well as physicians. In one randomized controlled study in Canada, Spitzer (1974) found no difference between NPs and physicians in the adequacy of their prescribing practices. More recently, data derived from log recordings of eighty-nine NPs in adult practice on 7,086 prescriptions showed drug utilization to be similar to physician prescribing, and intensity of prescribing to be less than that of physicians (Batey and Holland 1985). Physician consultation occurred in 14.3 percent of the prescriptions, mainly prior to prescribing for low-incidence conditions. Finally, a clinic study of over 2,000 decisions by NPs, conducted in 1985, found that physicians changed NP recommendations for over-the-counter medications and prescription drugs in only 2 percent of the cases (LaPlante and O'Bannon 1987).

With regard to the NP, some observers have suggested that the positive outcomes found are a result of the special way that this physician extender relates to patients. In recognizing the limits of the descriptive outcome studies, Sullivan (1982), in an editorial in the *American Journal of Public Health*, urged that a closer look be given to the nature of the interaction.

> Underlying explanations are hard to come by especially when the studies were to examine outcomes of treatment, and then only in relation to the specific diagnosis. These descriptive approaches are

Table 4.1

Equivalence in Quality of Care Provided by Nurse Practitioners (NPs) and Physicians (MDs), 1971–1986

Activity or measure	Setting	Study type
Process measures:		
Adequacy of pediatric physical assessment	Health center, low income neighborhood	Retrospective chart review
Adequacy of prescribing medication	Two MD family practice	Randomized controlled trial
Adequacy of the management of episodes of care	HMO	Prospective; chart review, timing of segments of patient visits
Management of hypertensive patients	Rural primary care center	Retrospective chart review
Similarity of treatment plan for pediatric patients	Military outpatient clinic	Retrospective evaluation of of NP's and MD's treatment plans
Short-and long-term compliance by patients	Emergency room	Prospective study with data collection at emergency room visit, followup
Outcome measures:		
Patient's physicial, emotional, and social functional status	Two MD family practice	Randomized controlled trial
Resolution of acute problems	Hospital ambulatory care clinics	Record review
Resolution of acute problems	Prepaid group practice	Survey of providers and patients with telephone followup of pts. at one week
Reduction in pain or discomfort among pediatric patients	Prepaid group practice	Survey as above

Source: U.S. Office of Technology Assessment. 1986. *Nurse Practitioners, Physician Assistants, and Certified Nurse-Midwives: A Policy Analysis.* Health Technology Case Study 37. Washington, D.C., Government Printing Office.

Table 4.2

Difference in Quality of Care Provided by Nurse Practitioners (NP) and Physicians (MD), 1974–1982

Activity or measure	Relative quality of care by NPs and MDs	Setting	Study Type
Process measure:			
Number of diagnostic tests	NP>MD	Hospital outpatient clinic	Random assignment of patients, record review, time and motion studies, patient interviews
Number of diagnostic tests	NP>MD	HMO	Prospective chart review, timing of segments of patient visits
Thoroughness of documentation of diagnosis and treatment information	NP> MD	Preventive medicine department of a multi-specialty clinic	Cross sectional: patient survey and chart review
Adequacy of telephone management of common pediatric problems	NP>MD	University pediatric clinic	Programmed calls from a trained person about selected pediatric problems; calls recorded and content analyzed

Table 4.2 Contd.

Activity or measure	Relative quality of care by NPs and MDs	Setting	Study Type
Effectiveness of interpersonal management skills (interviewing, communicating)	NP>MD	same as above	same as above
Management of problems requiring technical solutions	NP<MD	Jail health services	Review and audit
Outcome measures: Rate of patient return to employment	NP>MD	University hospital medical clinic	Random patient assignment: interviews, chart review
Reduction in number symptoms in patients	NP>MD	same as above	same as above
Level of patient awareness of provider orders	NP>MD	same as above	same as above
Level of control of blood pressure in patients with hypertension	NP>MD	City hospital and health department clinics	Record review
same as above	NP>MD	University hospital hypertension clinic	Prospective record review

Level of activity limitation and anxiety in patients with chronic problems	NP<MD	Prepaid group practice	Survey of providers and patients with telephone followup of pts. at one week
Amount of reduction of pain or discomfort in adult patients	NP>MD	same as above	same as above
Amount of weight reduction in obese patients	NP>MD	University hospital hypertension clinic	Prospective record review

Source: U. S. Office of Technology Assessment. 1986. *Nurse Practitioners, Physician Assistants, and Certified Nurse-Midwives: A Policy Analysis*. Health Technology Case Study 37. Washington, D.C., Government Printing Office.

necessary to examine the most basic questions of efficacy and safety of the nurse in comparison with other health workers; alternative designs, however, could show what nurses are doing to account for these changes and what interactions between nurse and client make for positive results. (Pp. 8–9)

Patient Satisfaction and the Management of Impressions

Americans view their health-care system, and their own health, largely as an extension of their highly individualistic, pragmatic, and technological orientation to the physical and social world. What people expect from health-care practitioners is derived in part from the values they want to maintain from what they have experienced in the past. David Mechanic (1972), in summarizing studies of health-care consumers, notes the common elements:

They seek to have a personal physician or a comparable source of care that is readily accessible to them and convenient to use. They want and expect their care to be competent, but they are equally concerned that those who provide it have an interest in them as people. They expect also that an adequate system of more specialized services will exist, if they should need them, and that they can obtain these services at a price that does not threaten them economically. (P. 2)

The capacity of the new health care practitioners to fit this description about what patients want depends not only on training and approval for exercising independent judgment but also can be an outcome of how their roles are defined. When they are permitted to carry their own caseload and follow patients on a long-term basis, they become the experts on those particular patients. Face-to-face contact is relatively frequent between any health-care practitioner and a patient when illness is being treated or monitored over a long duration. It follows that approval would be stronger where direct contact existed with physician extenders than where no contact existed. Furthermore, when NPs and PAs work with patients in dealing with emotional aspects of illness and health care, I would predict even greater approval, and little likelihood that patients will terminate contact or fail to take medications.

One of the most important explanations for the acceptance of PAs and NPs is their accessibility to patients. In the early days, Silver and Duncan (1971, 331–336) performed time-and-motion studies of the PNP, compared with office nurses and pediatricians, to determine whether the new practitioner created more opportunity for contact with patients. PNPs were found to spend twice as much time with patients as office nurses, with most of the contact in taking histories, performing physical examinations, evaluating health problems, and counseling parents. Other studies reported a reduction in the average time spent by the physician with the patient and family in pediatric private practices that employ nurse practitioners (Schiff, Fraser, and Walters 1969).

In many private practices and hospitals, standardized protocols are used by physician extenders in performing examinations or monitoring a treatment regimen. Protocols encourage a careful and systematic examination of the patient, making it incumbent on the examiner to perform tests when indicated by certain answers to questions. From the patient's perspective, the clearly observable use of the protocol may represent the presence of planning and technique, instilling confidence in the health-care organization.

Confidence can also be instilled in patients through the counseling and educational side of dispensing services. When dealing with chronically ill children or adults who need to be hospitalized periodically for treatment or diagnostic work, NPs and PAs are able to explain how to manage an illness at home or why one has to go to the hospital for surgical correction of a serious problem. In so doing, NPs and PAs can reduce the disruptive effects of being rehospitalized or discharged from the hospital. In their counseling and instructional efforts, physician extenders sometimes show how behavioral outbursts at home by a former patient are connected to a lengthy hospitalization or a fear of rehospitalization. This kind of preventive mental health work is usually done in consultation with a supervising physician, sometimes with psychiatrists or psychiatric social workers.

In the following exchange, recorded in my field notes, a PNP was able to explain to a child who had been subject to lengthy hospitalization for extensive reconstruction of his stomach that he was going to the hospital for a short-term visit, for an esophagram. Without this kind of preparation, the child might have believed that he was going into the hospital for a long stay.

> *PNP*: I have something to tell you, Fred. You can come to the hospital to play, not to stay. The doctors are going to take an X-ray. Do you know what X-rays are?
>
> *Fred*: X-rays?
>
> *PNP*: It's a picture. You have to drink something to make the picture work.

If patients do not wish to use a PA or NP, then it is very likely that the practitioner will not be employed to deliver primary care. For both PAs and NPs, the literature on patient acceptance is based on small samples of patients or their surrogates who use these services. By and large, the results suggest satisfaction with services delivered. Nontheless, occasional studies have found a reluctance on the part of patients to have either of these physician extenders perform independently as far as diagnostics and treatment are concerned (Smith 1981; Enggist and Hatcher 1983; Rodeghero 1978).

Experts on adult and pediatric practice have determined that from 60 to 80 percent of primary-care tasks can be delegated and can be performed without consultation. Therefore, when patients complain that an NP or PA is working independently, it is generally understood that they are not talking about procedures that go well beyond the ordinary practice. A person who believes that he or she can be helped only by a specialist may reject care from either a primary-care physician or a physician extender. Such patients usually see their problems as beyond the help of any primary-care provider.

All studies that examine the amount of time spent with patients found that PAs and NPs spend more time with patients than physicians do (Charney and Kitzman 1971; Health Services Research Center 1985; U.S. Congressional Budget Office 1979). While such studies have concluded that the output of NPs and PAs, as far as productivity is concerned, is not as great as that of physicians, the same data can also be used to suggest that the extra time spent by physician extenders with patients is perceived as a source of patient approval.

The more the patient sees the physician extender in the primary-care role, the higher the rate of acceptance (Linn 1976). In direct contact studies, patient approval for physician extenders has been very high, while mixed responses have been found when the public at large is asked about the wisdom of delegating various primary care medical tasks to NPs and PAs.

There have been several large-scale studies involving potential and actual consumers of physician-extender services carried out in different regions of the country. In a study based on 808 household interviews in Cuyahoga County, Ohio, Breslau and Novack (1979) found varied responses to the idea of delegating eighteen different medical tasks to nonphysician health workers.

Some of the variability in approval was based on how accessible existing providers were to the respondent. Any regular source of care might be better than none. In a large-scale rural study ($N = 3056$), researchers found more support for the role of nurse practitioner among young, low-income males when twelve medical functions were presented for possible delegation (Kviz, Misener, and Vinson 1983). Those who are especially dissatisfied with their usual source of health care are more likely to approve of task delegation.

In general, the public atmosphere appears to be one of acceptance (Hogan and Hogan 1982) . Older people, who currently have fewer barriers to care, owing to Medicare financing, are less likely to approve of the new health care practitioners because they see them as a substitute for their usual source of care. For the young, who may not always be insured, a potentially lower-cost provider enhances an inaccessible system of service (Fox and Storms 1980).

Several studies suggest that there are potential markets for nurse practitioners, even among affluent sectors of society, presumably those with a regular source of care. It is interesting to note that the organized world of nurse practitioners – the national associations – do not spend a great deal of time and energy on marketing; instead they demonstrate consumer interest and the feasibility of delivery of primary health-care services. In contrast, the new role of clinical pharmacy is heavily marketed as being cost effective (see Chapter 6).

While sample sizes are small, several studies in different areas of the country lead to the conclusion that among actual and potential consumers, there is widespread acceptance of the nurse practitioner. A New Haven study of 331 residents found that 62 percent of the respondents would use NP services. Dissatisfaction with present health care, family size, and age were the best predictors of intent to use services, provided they were covered by health insurance and if the costs were lower than physician care (Shamansky, Schilling, and Holbrook 1985). A Seattle study of 239 randomly selected respondents found potential users of family nurse practitioner services were likely to be women who are relatively more affluent, better-educated, and younger than the general population (Smith and Shamansky 1983). Finally, a cross-sectional survey of 388 residents of a northern Illinois county found that respondents who were favorable to prevention and health-promotion services — primarily the better educated — were also predisposed to use nurse practitioners, regardless of whether or not they had access to a regular personal physician (Pender and Pender 1980).

Despite these differences in outlook, many Americans now have heard of PAs and NPs. A telephone survey of 2,583 Baltimore urban households found that half the respondents had heard of these new roles in health care, but only 4 percent reported ever receiving care from an NP or PA. The sample members did not perceive any sharp differences between the two new health-care providers and respected the view that important primary-care functions could be delegated to physician extenders as long as they continued to report to the doctor (Storms and Fox 1979). In sum, physician extenders are no longer an innovation but are part of the organized world of health-care delivery. They are here to stay.

Some Anticipated and Unanticipated Problems

The public recognition of physician extender roles is matched by legislative ratification in forty-five states of the need to amend their nurse practices acts to make it possible for nurses to have an expanded role. By receiving legislative sanction to perform additional functions, NPs in the community can now enter into written agreements with physicians, who then oversee their work by reviewing patient records. This arrangement amounts to indirect supervision. Of particular concern in the review process is the quality of the work of NPs in making medical diagnoses and prescribing (Kolbert 1988, B2).

To what extent is this legal right to establish a community-based practice supported by professional associations in medicine and nursing? Interestingly, recent amendments to the New York State Nursing Practice Act, which would allow NPs (i.e., RNs with two additional years of training) to make some medical diagnoses and prescribe treatment in collaboration with physicians, was opposed by the major doctors' *and* nurses' organizations in the state. The state nursing association disapproved of making distinctions within nursing: (1) permitting those with more education to perform additional functions; and (2) implying that RNs who were not certified as NPs were not capable of diagnosing and treating illnesses (Kolbert 1988, B2). Nursing leaders were making the point that they believed all nurses could perform at that level of autonomy, and that more education and training would not make differentiation necessary. The Medical Society of New York State opposed the legislation on the grounds that it did not assure adequate supervision of physician extenders, despite the fact that NPs have to enter into a written agreement to have a physician review their patient records every three months.

The position of the New York State Nursing Association deserves comment. It is fair to say that professional associations do not like to see legal differentiations within their ranks. When practice rights are increased by statute, the professional association that represents the profession undergoing a collective mobility project wants to see all its professionals have their rights ratified at the same time. Legal distinctions in rank and responsibility lead to schisms and the formation of new organizations.

The medical profession's position is based more on strict marketplace considerations, given the increase in the number of doctors in the United States. The dominant profession's organized advocates do not want to see competition for the same (primary care) market and are particularly irritated when some of their brethren encourage it.

Role Expansion and Legal Problems

The faith of the state legislatures in the quality of the work of the NP has been borne out by the fact that there have been only two lawsuits in the United States in which NPs were co-defendents, based on their failure to diagnose correctly (Spitzer 1984, 1049). But the legal barriers to NPs have not been completely removed. And there continues to be *de facto* delegation of autonomy for some NPs. Regardless of enabling legislation, NPs have voluntarily reported that they write prescriptions and sign the name of the physician on the physician's prescription blank (Pearson 1986).

Once NPs work outside medical control, they may be seen as practicing medicine without a license. Going a kind of entrepreneurial route, NPs who set up independent practices have met with medical opposition in some states. Through lawsuits brought against nurse practitioners in Missouri, the state attorney general sought to get them to give up diagnosing and prescribing. The state court ruled that the nurses were practicing within an advanced or broad definition of nursing (Schwartz, deWolf, and Skipper 1987, 566). All acts performed by the NPs were deemed in accord with the state nurse practice act and were covered by the standing orders and protocols approved by physicians. The Missouri Supreme Court said:

> The hallmark of the professional is knowing the limits of one's professional knowledge. The nurse, either upon reaching the limit of her or his knowledge or upon reaching the limits prescribed for the nurse by the physician's standing orders and protocols, should refer the patient to the physician. (Quoted in Creighton 1984, 65)

In this case, there was no evidence to suggest that the nurses had exceeded these limits of clinical judgment. After this clear victory for NPs in Missouri, a similar lawsuit, brought by the Ohio Medical Board, and challenging the scope of nursing practice in that state, was dropped.

Concerning Direct Payment

With the establishment of Medicare and Medicaid, and the continued extension of medical benefits as an untaxed perquisite for employees and a tax deduction for employers, the question is raised concerning which professions are entitled to direct payment and which professions' services will be part of a total bill for services delivered by a provider, such as a hospital. The right to receive direct payment is extremely important for stabilizing the financial development of a profession. During the days of planning the 1965 social security legislation under which Medicare and Medicaid were financed, physicians who were delivering strictly technical services in hospitals (i.e., anesthesiologists, pathologists, and radiologists) fought strenuously to get their bills disaggregated from the total hospital bill. Without this achievement, their rates would be set by each hospital or would be determined by the overall per diem hospital rate, rather than by the "usual and customary" charges in the community. Independent billing meant that physicians who worked in hospitals could keep pace in their charges with the larger group of physicians who practiced in the community.

Direct payment or independent billing would make it possible for NPs to establish practices in the community to deliver their services in a way that would be administratively independent from a medical practice, but not clinically independent. Clinically, nurse practitioners and physician assistants can prescribe under standing orders or supervision by a physician. NPs can do this in eighteeen states in the union. Physicians can be reimbursed for these services by third-party payers, but physician extenders cannot, even when they perform exactly the same procedures. Clinically, physician extenders must be supervised when it comes to performing delegated medical tasks.

A second problem emerges when the tasks that PAs, and especially NPs, often do are examined as to whether they are covered by insurance. Health education and counseling, two major components of the role of the NP (and the PA), are not covered by most third-party payers. These nonprocedural services are vital in maintaining the health of patients or gaining their compliance with treatment regimens. Some HMOs employ NPs or PAs to perform many primary-care functions, including preventive ones, through education and counseling services.

By and large, third-party payers — a general term that refers to public insurers such as Medicare and Medicaid as well as profit-making and nonprofit insurance programs — have been very reluctant to honor claims for counseling and instructional services performed by nonphysicians. When they do pay for such services, they usually limit the number of consultations that can occur in the course of a single year, or there is a lifetime upper limit; sometimes, high deductibles and copayments are required.

The development of physician extenders as professions, particularly the NPs, is at a critical juncture. Approval by the medical establishment, even when there is a latent threat to medical hegemony, has been forthcoming in the two decades since the first NPs and PAs were trained. Tests of the ability of physician extenders to diagnosis and treat minor illnesses have been extensive, and practitioners compare favorably to physicians within their limited areas of competence. Public approval has also come about. Direct payment really depends on getting payers and group subscribers to see the value of consultation and educational services providing primary care, in managing chronic illness and preventing hospitalization. Managed care may be seen as cost saving by the insurance industry, and clearly the PA and the NP can be utilized as care managers as well as deliverers of primary care.

Alternatively, the rapid development of HMOs as a major source of comprehensive prepaid outpatient and inpatient medical care on a capitation basis, makes the employment of physician extenders, as the major in-house providers of primary care, a cost-effective policy for HMOs. Doctors who work in HMOs approve of this employment for NPs and prefer them to PAs.

In summary, helped along by their big brother (the profession of medicine), physician extenders have made substantial professional progress, receiving approval from doubting doctors and from patients who perceive them as accessible as well as capable. For NPs, the hurdle of independent billing and direct third-party reimbursement remains if they are to overcome financial limits on income imposed by administrative dependency on doctors. In contrast, as we see in the next chapter, clinical pharmacy has been making a wider effort to impress the public, with somewhat less success than among physician extenders.

References

Batey, M.V., and J.M. Holland. 1985. "Prescribing practices among nurse practitioners in adult and family health." *American Journal of Public Health* 75 (March): 258–262.

Breslau, N., and A.H. Novack. 1979. "Public attitudes toward some changes in the division of labor in medicine." *Medical Care* 17 (August): 859–867.

Brown, M.S. 1979. "Vantage point." *Nursing 79* (August): 78.

Burkett, G.L., and others. 1978. "A comparative study of physicians' and nurses' conceptions of the role of the nurse practitioner." *American Journal of Public Health* 68 (November): 1090–1096.

Charney, E., and H. Kitzman. 1971. "The child health nurse (pediatric nurse practitioner) in private practice: A controlled trial." *New England Journal of Medicine* 285 (December 9) : 1353–1358.

Claiborn, S.A., and W. Walton. 1979. "Pediatricians' acceptance of PNPs." *American Journal of Nursing* (February): 300.

Choi, M.W. 1981. "Nurses as co-providers of primary health care." *Nursing Outlook* (September): 519–521.

Creighton, Helen. 1984. "Law for the nurse manager: More about nurse practitioners." *Nursing Management* (September): 64–65.

Enggist, R.E., and M.E. Hatcher. 1983. "Factors influencing consumer receptivity to the nurse practitioner." *Journal of Medical Systems* 7 (December): 495–512.

Fowler, E.H. 1977. "Careers: Medical assistants—a new field." *New York Times* (July 6): D11.

Fox, J.G., and D.M. Storms. 1980. "New health practitioners and older persons." *Journal of Community Health* 5 (Summer): 244–253.

Greenberg, S. 1984. "On nonphysician 'associate residents.'" *New England Journal of Medicine* 311 (November 15): 1323.

Hanlon, C.R. 1980. "The surgeon's assistant: training and grammar." *Archives of Surgery* 115 (March) 243.

Health Services Research Center. 1985. *The National Rural Primary Care Evaluation Project: Issue-Oriented Data Analysis.* Chapel Hill, NC: University of North Carolina Press.

Hogan, K.A., and R.A. Hogan. 1982. "Assessment of the consumer's potential response to the nurse practitioner model." *Journal of Nursing Education* 21 (November): 4–12.

Johnson, R.E., and D.K. Freeborn. 1986. "Comparing HMO physician's attitudes toward NPs and PAs." *Nurse Practitioner* 11 (January): 39, 43–46, 49, et passim.

Kane, R.L. 1976. "Communication patterns of doctors and their assistants." *Medical Care* 14 (April): 348–356.

Kolbert, E. 1988. "Wider powers backed for nurse practitioners." *New York Times* (July 1): B2.

Kviz, F.J., T.R. Misener, and N. Vinson. 1983. "Rural health care consumers perceptions of the nurse practitioner role. *Journal of Community Health* 8 (Summer): 248–262.

Lamb, G.S., and R.J. Napodano. 1984. "Physician-nurse practitioner interaction patterns in primary care practices." *American Journal of Public Health* 74 (January): 26–29.

LaPlante, L.J., and F.V. O'Bannon. 1987. "NP prescribing recommendations." *Nurse Practitioner* 12 (April): 52–53, 57–58.

Lawrence, R.S., and others. 1977. "Physician receptivity to nurse practitioners: A study of the correlates of the delegation of clinical responsibility." *Medical Care* 15 (April): 298–310.

Levine, D.M. and others. 1976. "The role of new health practitioners in a prepaid group practice: Provider differences in process and outcomes of medical care." *Medical Care* 14 (April): 326–347.

Lewis, C.E., and T.K. Cheyovich. 1976. "Who is a nurse practitioner? Processes of care and patients' and physicians' perceptions." *Medical Care* 14 (April): 365–371.

Light, D.W. 1986. "Surplus versus cost containment: The changing context for health providers." In *Applications of Social Science to Clinical Medicine and Health Policy*, edited by Linda H. Aiken and David Mechanic, 519–542. New Brunswick: Rutgers University Press.

Linn, L.S. 1976. "Patient acceptance of the family nurse practitioner." *Medical Care* 14 (April): 357–364.

Little, M. 1980. "Nurse practitioner/physician relationships." *American Journal of Nursing* (September): 1040–1045.

Mechanic, David. 1972. *Public Expectations and Health Care: Essays on the Changing Organization of Health Services*. New York: Wiley Interscience.

Pearson, Linda, J. 1986. "NPs write prescriptions regardless of enabling legislation." *Nurse Practitioner* 11 (November): 6–7.

Pender, N.J., and A.R. Pender. 1980. "Illness prevention and health promotion services provided by nurse practitioners: predicting potential consumers." *American Journal of Public Health* 70 (November): 1204–1206.

Pierce, M., T.G. Quattlebaum, and J.B. Corley. 1985. "Significant attitude changes among residents associated with a pediatric nurse practitioner." *Journal of Medical Education* 60 (September): 712–718.

Robertson, W.J. 1983. "Nurse Practitioners and the Intensive Care Unit." *Pediatrics* 72 (August): 264–265.

Rodeghero, J.A. 1978. "Perceptions of nurse practitioners among the rural poor." *Nurse Practitioner* 3 (September/October): 7.

Scheffler, R.M. and D.B. Gillings. 1982. "Survey approach to estimating demand for physician assistants." *Social Science and Medicine* 16: 1039–1047.

Schiff, D.W., C.H. Fraser, and H.L. Walters. 1969. "The pediatric nurse practitioner in the office of pediatricians in private practice." *Pediatrics* 44 (July): 62–68.

Schwartz, H.D., P.L. deWolf, and J.K. Skipper. 1987. "Gender, professionalization and occupational anomie: The case of nursing." In *Dominant Issues in Medical Sociology*, edited by Howard D. Schwartz, 559–569. 2nd ed. New York: Random House.

Shamansky, S.L. , L.S. Schilling, and T.L. Holbrook. 1985. "Determining the market for nurse practitioner services: the New Haven experience." *Nursing Research* 34 (July-August): 242–247.

Silver, H.K., and B. Duncan. 1971. "Time-motion study of pediatric nurse practitioners: Comparison with regular office nurses and pediatricians." *Journal of Pediatrics* 79 (August): 331–336.

Silver, H.S., and P.A. McAtee. 1984. "On the use of nonphysician 'Associate Residents' in overcrowded specialty-training programs." *New England Journal of Medicine* 311 (August 2): 326–328.

Smith, C.W. 1981. "Patient attitudes toward physicians' assistants." *Journal of Family Practice* 13 (August): 201–204.

Smith, D.W., and S.L. Shamansky. 1983. "Determining the market for Family Nurse Practitioner services: the Seattle experience." *Nursing Research* 32 (September-October): 301–305.

Spitzer, W.O., and others. 1974. "The Burlington randomized trial of the nurse practitioner." *New England Journal of Medicine* 290 (January 31): 251–256.

Spitzer, Walter O. 1984. "The Nurse Practitioner revisited: The slow death of a good idea." *New England Journal of Medicine* 310 (April 19): 1049–1051.

Storms D.M., and J.G. Fox. 1979. "The public's view of physicians' assistants and nurse practitioners: a survey of Baltimore urban residents." *Medical Care* 17 (May): 526–535.

Sullivan, J.A. 1982. "Research on nurse practitioners: process behind the outcome?" *American Journal of Public Health* 72 (January): 8–9.

U.S. Congressional Budget Office. 1979. *Physician Extenders: Their Current and Future Role in Medical Care Delivery*. Washington, D.C.: Government Printing Office.

U.S. Office of Technology Assessment. 1986. *Nurse Practitioners, Physician Assistants, and Certified Nurse-Midwives: A Policy Analysis*. Health Technology Case Study 37. Washington, D.C.: Government Printing Office.

Vox Paed. 1978. "The case for pediatric nurse practitioners." *Clinical Pediatrics* 5 (May): 423–424.

Weiland, Anne P. 1983. "Physician and nurse joint practice: A description of nurse practitioners on a cardiac surgery service." *Heart and Lung* 12 (November) 576–580.

Chapter **5** Efforts to Change the Image of Pharmacy

When compared to physician extenders, clinical pharmacists live in a world of self-study and self-advocacy. Physician extenders are subject to study from external sources: Physicians, social scientists, and nurse researchers all want to show that the quality of care does not diminish with the use of NPs and PAs. And much of their product is directed toward the medical community, corporate rationalizers, and insurance companies.

In pharmacy, debates go on concerning not only whether pharmacy is changing but whether it should change. Advocates of clinical pharmacy, over a twenty-five-year period of editorializing in pharmacy journals, have sought to create a stronger sense of professionalism in the field. They want to find a new direction for a field that has lost its technical base and is threatened in community practice by chain store takeovers, leaving the community pharmacist in the position of being a hired hand. Moreover, employment in hospitals provides opportunities but also raises problems for the "patient oriented" pharmacist. This chapter identifies six themes, found in the writings of clinical pharmacy advocates, that would enable clinical pharmacy to break out of the fetters of the established profession: (1) identification of a new direction, (2) delegation of routine tasks, (3) need for continuing education, (4) avoiding false opportunities and seeking in-depth knowledge on pharmaceuticals, (5) raising the public image of practice and (6) increasing professionalism in the professional associations. Altogether, these themes constitute a strategy for the profession's mobility project. In essence, correct conduct is supposed to lead to institutional recognition in the health field and the autonomy in decision making found in medicine.

Pharmacy against Itself

In some ways, clinical pharmacy must stand apart from the very discipline it seeks to conquer. The demarcation of clinical pharmacy from other activities in the discipline—long a practical problem for professors of pharmacy and hospital pharmacists—is here examined as an *analytic* problem for sociologists of professions. Although the construction of a boundary between clinical pharmacy and traditional pharmacy is useful for the clinical pharmacists' pursuit of professional goals, particularly the acquisition of cultural authority and the opportunity to practice clinical pharmacy, it is only one of several mechanisms by which an established profession seeks to change its position within a single industry.

I have identified the traditional style of professional development via internal ethical reform along with a more rigorous education (Birenbaum 1982) as insufficient to produce career opportunities for clinical pharmacists. Internal reform puts the emphasis on professionalism, a characteristic of the provider of a service, which is not the same thing as empowerment of the profession, what Eliot Freidson (1970) referred to as "professionalization." Building on this analysis, we can inquire whether it is necessary to the quest for upgrading to go beyond developing a more consistent professional image, to find (1) markets for services, while creating (2) cognitive creditability within the health care field, and standardizing (3) the production of trained clinicians, subjects to which I turn in the two chapters that follow.

It is useful to consider improvement of professional image as part of a collective social mobility project. Larson (1977) states that the success of a profession's organizational efforts determines whether mobility is going to occur. More than striving, this effort must be cooperative among those who are similarly situated. Creating a consistent image becomes a central task to accomplish in order to gain public and professional support for a collective mobility project.

Creating a consistent image of a profession is "identity work," requiring the development of uniformity in the behavior and attitude of members, no small task to accomplish in a complex society. Yet to get others to give pharmacists respect, and the opportunities to be autonomous and responsible, requires the remaking of professional activity. Consistency in behavior and attitude become prerequisites for the remaking of a profession:

> Unlike craft or industrial labor most professions produce intangible goods: their product, in other words, is only formally alienable and is inextricably bound to the person and the personality of the producer. It follows therefore, that *the producers themselves have to be produced* if their products or commodities are to be given a distinctive form. (Larson 1977; italics in original)

If Larson's hypothesis is correct, then a crucial development that makes professional autonomy possible is a focus on the *performers* of the tasks rather than the performance (i.e, that they are imbued with the appropriate qualities). To what extent is such a set of activities evident in the profession of pharmacy? Gieryn, Bevins, and Zehr (1985, 393) have noted that aspiring professions seek to construct social boundaries as a way of marketing their services. This is another way of talking about "identity work," according to tensions and strains between representatives of different knowledge-based providers of services. Arguing that these social boundaries enhance professionalization, the authors assert (1) that boundaries create demand for a distinctive commodity and (2) boundaries serve to exclude providers of "similar" services (Gieryn, Bevins, and Zehr, 1985, 393).

Boundary work could conceivably be aimed by advocates of clinical pharmacy at competitors among physicians and nurses' concern with improving patient compliance and preventing adverse drug interactions. But this is not the case, since adverse drug interactions seems to be of little concern in other health professions. As we see in chapter 6, some of the work of the reform movement in pharmacy has been aimed at gaining respect from these segments of other professions.

Marketing clinical pharmacy has not been a fully successful collective mobility project for the reform minded in the profession. Pharmacy has an image problem—a direct result of the public's perception of the pharmacist as the ally of the drug manufacturer (Dichter 1973). As a purveyor of pharmaceuticals, the pharmacy profession is dismissed as commercially minded, an evaluation that threatens the professional collective mobility project of clinical pharmacists. Moreover, the problems faced by the clinical movement involve not only the public but the medical profession as well, a market for services that surely must be won over if reprofessionalization is to succeed. The situation is confused and confusing not only because of the structural differentiation of the profession but also because of a lack of agreement on purpose among its members.

The War of Words in Pharmacy

The central tensions as well as aspirations of an occupation in contemporary society are found in the publications for practitioners of the craft. Covering a thirty year period, all of the major journals in pharmacy were examined to locate articles, editorials, and letters that dealt with questions and issues related to professional behavior, aspirations and organizational goals. These statements are the data utilized to understand how advocates of reprofessionalization have shaped the strategies for improving the image of pharmacy. Less systematic efforts were made to identify similar materials in other journals in the health-care field. No interviews were conducted with advocates of clinical pharmacy because it was reasoned that their public statements combined their response to strains within the field and efforts to promote their interests (Gieryn 1983).

Pharmacy does not seem to want to step on the territory of medicine. Unlike new tasks acquisitions that would change the boundaries of pharmacy, these activities call for status-ratifying activities on the part of significant others and few transfers of cultural authority.

Image Changing Activities

Identification of a New Direction

Given the often mentioned "crisis of purpose" in pharmacy, and its uneven commitment to a clinical professional role in health care, a collective mobility drive starts with restating the purpose of pharmacy in a way that attempts to speak for all its members, a technique often associated with groups that are seeking to change their position in society. While not all pharmacists would agree, clinical advocates claim that the purpose of contemporary pharmacy is the advancement of rational drug therapy. This purpose can be obtained in the long run only if the major training facilities — the colleges of pharmacy — agree that this is their primary mission. And this mission can be accomplished by producing a patient-oriented pharmacist.

An independent professional, however, has to know what other professions can and cannot do in the health-care system. Therefore, the production of patient-oriented pharmacists cannot take place in separate educational programs but only in cooperative and integrated academic surrounds, where physicians, nurses, and other health care providers are educated and trained. In this way, pharmacists can learn not only what others do but can demonstrate what *they* can do in performing specific health care functions (Provost 1971c). In this manner, pharmacists receive legitimation as players on the health care team, an important basis for marketing their skills.

An active professional has to receive the best training and not settle for minimum standards of competency. Consequently, the patient-oriented pharmacist will inevitably be the recipient of the Pharm.D. degree, the clinical movement's proposed initial degree of entry into the profession. Understandably, currently practicing pharmacists are somewhat resistant to this objective, for there are substantial differences in the educational attainments of registered pharmacists, trained at different times and practicing under varying state legislation.

Delegation of Routine Tasks

An upgraded educational requirement for pharmacists is considered highly desirable by some pharmacists, but it is also recognized that an image change comes from other sources. Zellmer (1977) states that "the status of practice is shaped by routine functions of the majority of pharmacists and by perceptions of the public" (p.929). The pharmacy college, however, is regarded as the major force for improving the profession's overall level of service, implying that new technical training programs must be created under its auspices. Pharmacy colleges are exhorted to implement the training for a new division of labor, a distribution of tasks in such a way that the pharmacist will have a managerial role. Colleges must have immediate concern for the training of personnel to perform pharmacy's basic drug distribution and control functions. To a large extent, these basic functions can be executed most efficiently by trained technical personnel supervised by pharmacists. Therefore, fewer pharmacists and many more technicians should be trained (Zellmer 1977).

Clearly, the advocates for restructuring the mission of colleges of pharmacy are emulating the corporate rationalizers of the health-care system (Alford 1972). A rational drug therapy requires a rational allocation of personnel. The technical functions of pharmacists of the past, and of many pharmacists in current practice, will become functions of the pharmacy technician of the future. The pharmacist of the future must have knowledge as well as administrative skills in order to be able to assume new roles.

The Need for Continuing Education

The role of drug expert and clinical coordinator of the patient's rational drug therapy must continue to grow and change. Continuing education is needed to make this possible. Part of the process of upgrading pharmacy and producing new professionals involves mandatory continuing education, and some states have already adopted such requirements. While older pharmacists often find these educational programs burdensome and boring, younger members of the profession are appalled at the disrespect shown by their elders for learning. Some members of the profession are not interested in upgrading their knowledge and skills, since it will not necessarily mean greater responsibility or increased compensation for performing new tasks. Some states have further broken down the continuing education requirements for relicensing into different programs for institutional and community pharmacists (Angorn 1972).

Rationality in the profession does not stop with creating a new division of labor and system of education. Advocates of the clinical role have called for further steps to ensure uniformity in training, seeking to create consistent requirements among the states and a single national standard for accreditation of continuing education (Provost 1972). Interestingly, some hospital pharmacy units have become education oriented on their own, independent of state requirements, and have adopted in-house education programs (Jeffrey and Gallina 1974). Hospital pharmacists have also sought to educate nurses and physicians through the development of an institution-wide bulletin on drugs.

Avoiding False Opportunities and Seeking In-Depth Knowledge

Doing for others, or better, guarding the welfare of others, is the ideal abstract purpose of the professions. Clinical pharmacy attempts to maintain this ideal and extend it to everyone in the profession. A consistent professional image requires methods of maintaining a favorable public impression, particularly when pharmacists attempt to perform patient-oriented roles. There must be a developed commitment to service, and a sense of responsibility, identified by Freidson (1970) as professionalism, and a sense of mutual dependence on one's peers for standards of behavior and evaluation. One way to maintain and convey a professional image is to turn down opportunities for any role expansion that ultimately may do harm to the patient. When health planners advocated that the pharmacist be trained in primary care, much in the same way that physician extenders are employed, the *American Journal of Hospital Pharmacy* took a guarded view of this proposal, claiming that this new role should be considered from the vantage point of what is good for the patient, not from the collective standpoint that the pharmacist is overtrained and underutilized (Provost 1971b).

In sticking to what they know, pharmacists are genuinely expected to make a lasting impression on significant others, using their expertise to solve problems, and in turn producing opportunities for purposeful role expansion. The temptations of role expansion are many, but clinical pharmacy leaders seek to get pharmacy to stick to its true purpose. At the same time, effective clinical pharmacists know in what areas of health care their services are and are not distinctive and valued. To achieve genuine results, one has to consider not only the patient's best interest but to convince the powers that be of one's commitment.

The rejection of primary-care roles is not based on a complete unwillingness to take on a subordinate role. Francke (1972) sought to build a bridge to clinical pharmacology, a field of medicine in which practitioners were in short supply. In making the offer (in a medical journal) to become the applied side of this medical specialty, clinical pharmacist Francke acknowledged that his profession would benefit from association with physicians: "the clinical pharmacist can monitor adverse effects of drugs and conduct drug utilization studies throughout the hospital; he would receive much more cooperation with these activities if he were associated with a clinical pharmacologist" (Francke 1972, 387).

A purposeful rationality accompanies the emphasis found earlier on developing a new division of labor. Much in the manner of true believers, pharmacists will make a lasting impression on the skeptics or, in this case, the disbelieving world around them.

> Armed with either the appropriate academic credentials or self-acquired knowledge, they expand their responsibilities by thoroughly documenting and evaluating their performance in a new area. Using this evidence to bolster their credibility, they integrated these innovations into routine practice and occasionally, enveloped areas that were once the exclusive territory of other professions or disciplines. (Tally 1980, 641)

In attempting to maintain the evangelical spirit and dedication of clinical pharmacy, the writer of the above is equally fearful of mock clinicians in pharmacy as resistance from the outside. Facile solutions are not going to do the movement any good. Pharmacists are essentially warned not to get in over their heads when they seek to solve problems "without solid development of the skills required" (Tally 1980, 641). True professionalism, he states, is based on a recognition of where to learn something, and this learning may come from interprofessional dialogue as well as academic credentials. Others have suggested that pharmacists who are unwilling to learn new things or are incompetent should be driven from the bosom of the profession (Tally 1980, 641).

Only those who know can practice, say the leaders; and the systematic acquisition of knowledge becomes the foundation for its institutional use. The acquisition of theory and method is recognized by clinical advocates as the precious source of repro-fessionalization. Brodie (1981) calls for a new theoretical base for pharmacy, while Watanabe and his associates (1975) proffer a systematic approach to drug information requests, in essence a way or organizing a professional response to the problems of others. But pharmacists also need opportunities to display what they can do, and the various hospital standing bodies, such as Drug Use Review and Institutional Review Committees, become showcases for the new pharmacists (Tremblay 1981; Raehl, Miller, and Foster 1981).

Advocates claim that success will not come merely through being a drug expert. The importance of the contribution of a drug information specialist is central in establishing a rational policy in hospitals. But the drug intelligence function must be matched by skills in patient care. The pharmacist-patient rela-tionship involves the development of communication skills (Ivey, Tso, and Stamm 1975; Smith 1977). If the relationship between pharmacist and patient is upgraded to more than a casual or fleet-ing encounter, then new issues arise concerning the *right* of a patient to choose a clinical pharmacist. Clinical pharmacists do not see themselves as freestanding professionals, however. Since they are employed primarily in HMOs and hospitals, the issue of choice is dismissed by advocates of the clinical role for pharmacists. Still, the emergence of an issue of this kind offers advocates another opportunity to remind people that they are interested solely in the welfare of the patient rather than in preserving traditional relationships and values. More concretely, the parallel is drawn with the anesthesiologist, radiologist, and pathologist — all physicians who serve the patient under the coordinating physician's direction — who are not selected by the patient (Smith 1977, 33). An additional parallel is suggested: The clinically oriented would like to acquire the billing rights now enjoyed by these three medical specialties, as well as find a niche for themselves in organized health care. Virtue is not just its own reward.

Raising the Public Image of the Profession

Careful efforts have been made by reformers to change the image of pharmacy, but what have been the results of this campaign? A 1974 national survey conducted for the Food and Drug Administration found that few physicians rated the pharmacist very highly as a source of drug information (Applied Management Sciences 1974). Physicians at that time (and maybe forever) consulted other physicians, and even detail men, more frequently than pharmacists when seeking drug information; they also rated colleague physicians, detail men, and outside physician consultants as more useful contacts than contacts with pharmacists. The 10,000 physicians surveyed sought to have an impartial, university trained, and employed detail man assist them in gaining drug information, a role that the advocates of change within pharmacy insist that pharmacists can play. No significant percentage of the sample suggested that pharmacists perform this role. The clinically oriented are not dismayed by these findings and insist that the opinion of physicians can be changed.

Founders of the clinical movement are somewhat more pessimistic about the capacity of the public to reconsider the profession. They are extremely sensitive to the popular image of pharmacy, as based on the retail drug store. Articles and editorials, starting in the 1960s, have called for the separation of pharmacies and drug stores (Francke 1969). Control over the profession has been seen as in the hands of chain-store owners, often conglomerates, and pharmacists who own drug stores; while 62 percent of community pharmacists are employees (Millis 1975). Many of the employed are recent graduates and are motivated to change the community pharmacy practice environment (Zellmer 1977, 929).

This situation is encouraging to reformers, who seek to reach the powerless employee in community pharmacy. By changing the *producers* of the product (the prescription), the clinically oriented seek to raise professional and ethical issues in community pharmacy, thus organizing the unorganized in commercial settings. Advocates of reprofessionalization in community pharmacy call for total separation, both legally and organizationally, of the pharmacy and the drug store. Arriving at professional performance requires the acquisition of legal rights to restrict pharmacy and ethical codes that would interdict commercialism. In setting apart the pharmacy from the drug store, reformers would legally restrict pharmacists from practicing in any commercial enterprise, including registered pharmacists who owned such stores. Just as the doctor has an office with examining facilities and consultation rooms, the pharmacist would prepare a proper workplace. Producing the ways in which the professionals manage impressions of themselves, it can be said, is equally as important to the collective mobility project as the production of competent professionals.

The capacity of the public to recognize the changing role of the pharmacist is considered to be very limited. After all, does the public really care to call into being yet another clinical profession, pay more for what appears to be the same services, and have to show deference to a new hierarchically oriented group? The profession of pharmacy is so unevenly developed that it is hard for the consumer to identify a clinical contribution. Moreover, there is no unified group with closed ranks to impress the public. Aside from the structural side of pharmacy, there is also the question of its social purpose, which is not very visible outside the pharmacy journals.

It has often been said that professions make claims to be public service minded. It is hard to see which claims are real and which are false. Air traffic controllers, for example, threatened to strike in 1981 over issues of work schedules that they claimed threatened the safety of the flying public. The federal Department of Transportation denied that the work was as stressful as workers claimed. Here the profession was not considered capable of making a judgment about its own work. The work performed by air traffic controllers may be stressful, and they are responsible for the lives of passengers, but the profession has not established a right to make the judgment when the health and safety of the public is affected by their schedules. Physicians, in contrast, can declare public health emergencies. Salaried physicians, as in

England's National Health Service, are represented by medical associations that bargain collectively with the government ministry concerning their workload. They have a great deal to say about what is a safe patient panel, one that will give them sufficient time to devote to patient needs.

Pharmacy is still not seen as dealing with problems of this magnitude or drama. Clinical pharmacists have called for a public relations campaign to communicate "the profession's social policies and action to the public so as to gain its good will" (Zellmer 1972, 119). The consumer is invited to sit on boards of national pharmacy organizations for educational purposes: "It cannot be assumed that the public understands and appreciates pharmacy's policies and deeds. Clinical pharmacists want to make it clear that they are not in the keep of the drug industry" (Ruggiero 1973, 312). Further, they wish to protect the public's wealth by calling for generic substitution of prescribed drugs, where appropriate, a procedure that could save money for patients or third-party payers (Provost 1967).

The public image, to the dismay of reformers, is based on the statistical norm in pharmacy practice rather than the exemplary few. A single national organization is conceded to be desirable for improving the image of American pharmacy. Unity gives pharmacists the image of strength, but, it is argued, this solidarity has to be based on the overall consistency of practitioners.

> Before there can be meaningful organizational unity, there must be de facto unity at the practice level. This de facto unity would be demonstrated by a prevailing commitment among practitioners to principles of professional service. (Zellmer 1978, 1041)

Increasing Professionalism in the Associations

The image of professional societies is equally inconsistent, according to internal critics of pharmacy. These organizations are castigated for producing poor-quality publications that are merely vehicles for heavy pharmaceutical advertising. The editorializing of the *American Journal of Hospital Pharmacy* (*AJHP*) suggests that the policy of this journal is somewhat more restrictive of advertising. In twice reviewing their policy in the 1970s, the claim was made that the *AJHP* strictly limited advertising copy to that which preserved the principles of pharmaceutical ethics and effective practices. The American Society of Hospital Pharmacists specifically excluded advertisements that offered gratuities and inducements to pharmacists (ASHP Board 1972). Manufacturing practices were investigated by the society before the journal accepted ads from pharmaceutical houses (Editorial 1977). In general, the journal demanded a scientific content to its articles and held to strict ethical standards when it came to advertising. In reflecting on its policies, editor Provost (1966) held to the position that the *AJHP* was aimed at the clinically oriented.

Critical comments were made by the *AJHP* editor about journals published by state associations of pharmacists. After determining that the quality of original articles published in state journals was poor, this clinical pharmacy advocate also suggested that the policy of republishing useful articles from other journals was an unnecessary contribution to the profession. He concluded that state association journals were an embarrassment to the profession, containing pharmaceutical advertising and little else, and being one reason "why pharmacy is held in rather low regard by its sister professions and by the public" (Provost 1971a, 153).

While every profession has its journals, pharmacy was seen to have an extremely large number. According to the *Pharmaceutical Director*, an American Pharmaceutical Association publication, the field contains 113 national, regional, state, and local publications. The range in quality is undoubtedly great, but can one argue that pharmacy is any different from other clinical professions where drugs and equipment are marketed through the practitioner? The profession of medicine has an equally great range in quality in its journals, and many doctors refer to unsolicited journals they receive as "throwaways."

Professionalism and Reprofessionalization

It is noteworthy that reformers in pharmacy are extremely sensitive to their public image as a profession, believing that a reduction in the number of professional journals as well as other efforts, are required to improve the image. The concern for quality by the avatars of clinical pharmacy reveals an effort to match or outdo their sister professions, perhaps overconforming to the norms of clinical science. The purification of the profession, in word as well as deed, becomes the method of arriving at clinical responsibilities. Perhaps an effort to embrace the statistical norm in the journal arena will help to improve the overall quality of written materials, and in so doing, disarm critics rather than create antagonists.

Outreach efforts have been attempted by reformers in the community. In a movement led by university-based teachers and clinicians who stress ethical and scientific standards in health care, there is a great gap between the garden-variety community pharmacist and the clinically oriented. Effort and communication are required on the part of the true believers to improve the community pharmacist's skills and image. Community pharmacists are perceived as wanting to act more professionally, and are advised to do so in occasional articles that appear in the commercially oriented *American Druggist* or *Contemporary Pharmacy Practice* (Robbins 1977; Puckett and others 1978).

A concern for image is found among all workers, and in this case it is only part of an effort by clinical pharmacists to convince physicians, hospital administrators, and the public that they provide necessary services. These efforts in some ways contradict the self-admitted capacity of pharmacists for passivity, for the clinically oriented need to prove, according to the norms of research and evaluation, the value of their contribution to increasing patient compliance with drug treatment regimens. Science, as a method of persuasion, undoubtedly receives a great deal of respect in the health-care world, even when used by lower-status occupations such as pharmacy.

A great deal of the effort to reprofessionalize in pharmacy is based on an inward-looking focus on increasing professionalism. Needed, in addition, are opportunities to reward members of the profession through clinical practice (Birenbaum 1982). The dilemma for the leadership of the clinical pharmacy movement is how to increase the status of the profession while gaining more cultural authority. Either course is likely to produce conflict. Some of the status-enhancing activities advocated in the professional literature effectively separate clinical pharmacists from pharmacists in retail endeavors. The role-expanding activities undertaken challenge the monolithic authority of physicians in the area of patient care. How these conflicts are resolved will determine whether the effort to reprofessionalize will reach the objectives desired by advocates of clinical pharmacy. Surely a new image will emerge, but one that is hardly likely to be consistent with the goal of unified profession.

References

Alford, R.R. 1972. "The political economy of health care: Dynamics without change." *Politics and Society*: 127–164.

Angorn, R.A. 1972. "The Florida 'institutional pharmacy' law." *American Journal of Hospital Pharmacy* 29: 970–972.

Applied Management Sciences. 1974. *Survey of Drug Information Needs and Problems Associated with Communications Directed to Practicing Physicians. Part 1; Physician Information Survey.* Washington, D.C.: Food and Drug Administration.

American Society of Hospital Pharmacists (ASHP) Board. 1972. "Statement of advertising policy of the American Society of Hospital Pharmacists." *American Journal of Hospital Pharmacists* 30: 621.

Birenbaum, A. 1982. "Reprofessionalization in Pharmacy." *Social Science and Medicine* 16: 871–878.

Brodie, D.C. 1981. "Need for a theoretical base for pharmacy practice." *American Journal of Hospital Pharmacy* 38: 49–54.

Dichter Institute. 1973. *Communicating the Value of Comprehensive Pharmaceutical Services to the Consumer.* Washington, D.C.: American Pharmaceutical Association.

Editorial. 1977. "Advertising in the journal." *American Journal of Hospital Pharmacy* 34: 1191.

Francke, D.E. 1969. "Let's separate pharmacies and drugstores." *American Journal of Hospital Pharmacy* 141: 161–176.

_____. 1972. "The relationship between clinical pharmacology and clinical pharmacy." *The Journal of Clinical Pharmacy* 12: 384–392.

Freidson, E. 1970. *The Profession of Medicine: A Study of the Sociology of Applied Knowledge.* New York: Dodd, Mead.

Gieryn, T.F., G.M. Bevins, and S.C. Zehr. 1985. "The professionalization of american scientists." *American Sociological Review* 50: 392–408.

Gieryn, T.F. 1983. "Boundary-work and the demarcation of science from non-science: Strains and interests in professional ideologies of scientists." *American Sociological Review* 48: 781–795.

Ivey, M., Y. Tso, and K. Stamm. 1975. "Communication techniques for patient instruction." *American Journal of Hospital Pharmacy* 32: 828–831.

Jeffrey, L.P., and J.N. Gallina. 1974. "Pharmacist standard for maintaining professional competence." *American Journal of Hospital Pharmacy* 31:943–946.

Larson, M. 1977. *The Rise of Professionalism: A Sociological Analysis.* Berkeley: University of California.

Millis, J. 1975. *Pharmacists for the Future: The Report of the Study Commission on Pharmacy.* Ann Arbor: Health Administration Press.

Provost, G.P. 1966. "For the masses of the few?" *American Journal of Hospital Pharmacy* 23: 331.

_____. 1967. "The AMA and generic prescribing." *American Journal of Hospital Pharmacy* 24: 103.

_____. 1971a. "State pharmaceutical journals: Legitimate need or ego fulfillment?" *American Journal of Hospital Pharmacy* 28: 153.

_____. 1971b. "The pharmacist as a primary practitioner: A guarded view." *American Journal of Hospital Pharmacy* 28: 239.

_____. 1971c. "Considerations in clinical pharmacy education and practice." *American Journal of Hospital Pharmacy* 28: 841.

_____. 1972. "On the concept of free choice of pharmacy." *American Journal of Hospital Pharmacy* 29: 33.

Puckett, F.J., and others. 1978. "Pharmacist patient counseling practices." *Contemporary Pharmacy Practice* 1: 67–71.

Raehl, C.L., D.E. Miller, and T.S. Foster. 1981. "Pharmacist involvement in institutional review of clinical trials." *American Journal of Hospital Pharmacy* 38: 334–339.

Robbins, J. 1977. "Pharmacy's unfullfilled status as a profession." *American Druggist* 176: 34, 37.

Ruggiero, J.S. 1973. "Clinical pharmacy and the pharmaceutical industry." *American Journal of Hospital Pharmacy* 30: 311–315.

Smith, M.D. 1977. "Management of the pharmacist–patient relationship strategy using sociological concepts." *Journal of the American Pharmaceutical Association* 17: 761–763.

Tally, C. R. 1980. "Those faking pharmacists." *American Journal of Hospital Pharmacy* 37: 641.

Tremblay, J. 1981. "Creating an appropriate climate for drug use review." *American Journal of Hospital Pharmacy* 38: 212–215.

Watanabe, A.S., and others. 1975. "Systematic approach to drug information requests." *American Journal of Hospital Pharmacy* 32: 1282–1285.

Zellmer, W.A. 1972. "Pharmacy and the public interest." *American Journal of Hospital Pharmacy*: 29: 119.

_____. 1977. "Efforts of upgraded pharmacy education on pharmacy practice." *American Journal of Hospital Pharmacy* 34: 929.

_____. 1978. "Unity in pharmacy." *American Journal of Hospital Pharmacy* 35: 1041.

Chapter 6

**Cultural Authority and
Boundary Work: Creating
Markets For Clinical Pharmacy**

The sociological study of the rise of professionalism (Larson 1977) and professional autonomy (Starr 1982) as features of modern society has identified a model that new professions, and old ones as well, seek to follow. In particular, professions that seek to upgrade their position in a division of labor must work constantly at distinguishing themselves from more traditional and circumscribed practitioners.

An example of this effort is found in an unwitting comparison, as well as a definition, by two sociologists writing about drug iatrogenesis as a social problem. Claiming that clinical pharmacy was developed to reduce instances of adverse drug effects due to prescription errors by physicians, the authors also legitimate clinical pharmacy's social purpose:

> Called "clinical pharmacy," this role is a transformation of pharmacists' traditional responsibilities for the safe storage, distribution and accurate dispensing of drugs prescribed by physicians. In the discharge of such core activities — which are said to be "product focused" — pharmacists also find themselves in the position of serving as information providers and drug consultants to both physicians and patients. The provision of such information is the essence of clinical pharmacy and, as a cluster of activities, it is said to be "patient-focused." These consultations are seen as clinical because they require pharmacists to be knowledgeable about and directly involved in reviewing patients' medical histories and ongoing treatments. (Broadhead and Facchinetti 1985, 425)

The demarcation of clinical pharmacy from other activities in the discipline involves the construction of a boundary between clinical pharmacy and traditional pharmacy practices. It is a useful accomplishment for clinical pharmacists in their pursuit of professional goals, particularly the acquisition of cultural authority and opportunities to practice clinical pharmacy; but it is only one of several mechanisms by which an established profession seeks to change its position within a single industry. Building on this model of professionalization, we can inquire whether or not it is necessary to the quest for upgrading also to (1) create markets for services as well as (2) develop a more consistent professional image, (3) create cognitive creditability within the health care field, and then (4) standardize the production of trained clinicians. This chapter explores recent efforts undertaken by advocates of clinical pharmacy in the United States to create stable markets. My purpose is to advance theoretical understanding concerning the origins and outcomes of movements to upgrade a profession, as well as to understand the tensions that exist within an internally autonomous but dependent profession that stands in the shadow of medicine.

It is useful to consider the acquisition of markets as part of a collective upward mobility project, not just as a way of increasing remuneration for pharmacy services. The movement toward increased cultural authority and career opportunities involves what may be regarded as positioning the product among competing products. Alternatively, the organized efforts engaged in by advocates of upgrading the profession may be termed "boundary work" (Gieryn 1983, 781–795). This analysis identifies instances in which advocates of clinical pharmacy use others as a foil to promote their case for greater recognition. Gieryn (1983) hypothesizes that "when the goal is *expansion* of authority or expertise into domains claimed by other professions or occupations, boundary-work heightens the contrast between rivals in ways flattering to the ideologist's side" (pp. 791–792; italics in original).

Beyond boundary work are the methods of persuading those in important positions that the services available are useful and that the profession deserves recognition. Inducing major decision makers and the public to use a service helps create predictable markets and is a way of achieving recognition as a cultural authority. It is important to understand how these efforts are conducted. Any profession may contain seemingly contradictory goals, technologies, and norms. Pharmacy is more than full of such contradictions; it is very much a profession undergoing serious internal transformations, perhaps even fissions.

As in the previous chapter, I have used the writings in pharmacy journals over the past twenty-five years that seek to promote greater acquisition of stable sources of clinical activities. Advocates of clinical pharmacy are seeking to perform activities deemed important in patient care management (Fletcher 1978; Nardone, Reuler, and Girard 1980; Platt 1981; Pendleton, Brouwer, and Jaspers 1983; Platt and McMath 1979). It is apparent that the clinical content of the objectives of reformers in pharmacy overlaps with concerns expressed in medicine about the need to improve provider-patient communication and medication compliance (Haynes, Taylor and Sackett 1979). Guidelines for interviewing have been elaborated in great detail by physicians, starting with how to begin a consultation (Reiser and Schroder 1980). Furthermore, the clinical communication process has been linked in studies to patient compliance or adherence to medical prescriptions; to the number of medication errors made by a patient; and to failures to keep appointments (Carter and others 1982, 550). Pendleton (1983) has recently reviewed numerous studies on patient satisfaction, as well as less frequently found studies that relate social behavioral variables to compliance.

The complexity of modern treatment regimens has been associated with reduced patient compliance with them (Becker 1985). In response to these findings, instruction and reassurance of patients concerning their treatment regimens have been attempted by other health-care providers besides physicians. Nurses have become involved in managing patient compliance with medication regimens (Marston 1977). And impressive empirical support has been found for involving pharmacists in similar work (Schwartz 1976; Sharpe 1977; Hartoum and others, 1986).

Clearly efforts are being made to have patients understand their treatment regimens and to improve patient compliance with them by many professions in health care. Only within pharmacy has a segment sought to organize an entire profession around these objectives, focusing on enhancing the effectiveness and safety of drug therapy. And it should be said that this effort is associated mainly with hospital-based and younger pharmacists, rather than with that part of the profession in retail situations.

Expanding the Boundaries of Pharmacy

The first step in making pharmacy a clinical profession was the development of concepts that could be implemented to protect the patient's health while giving pharmacists more responsibility and interaction with physicians and nurses. Clinical pharmacy, an idea now widely accepted in the profession, was defined in an editorial in the publication that provided the cutting edge for the movement, the *American Journal of Hospital Pharmacy (AJHP)*. Not merely the drug provider, the clinical pharmacist now would be engaged in promoting safety and effectiveness in drug use (Provost 1971, 77). Despite this clear definition of a complex task, Provost went on to assert that in the future, pharmacy would no longer need this "clinical" label, or any other, provided that the profession "embraces the opportunity to offer services distinguished from other parts of pharmacy" (p.77). In other words, in the future, all pharmacists, including those in the community, would be professionally engaged in clinical practice.

The major activities involved in a segment of a profession seeking to expand its responsibilities and rewards are identified as (1) creating awareness of a service, (2) restrictions on practice, (3) upgrading of responsibilities, (4) client remuneration for upgraded activities, (5) aggressive marketing of services, and (6) innovative projects.

Creating Awareness of a Service

The *AJHP* in 1981 published an article advocating the use of marketing concepts in order to gain acceptance of clinical pharmacy in hospitals (Grauer 1983). Ironically, the marketing of clinical pharmacy in practice had been proceeding for fifteen years, both in intentional and unwitting ways. In advancing the cause of clinical pharmacy, its advocates called for the development of methods that would establish expectations for these services in consumers so that they would become dependent on them. These expectations need a great deal of changing. Physicians, in particular, are a group that could use these new expectations; in 1966, the *AJHP* published an article by a physician (Keefer 1966) on his sources of drug information that never mentioned the pharmacist as a source!

Marketing an occupational specialty often means breaking down reliance on alternative means of receiving services, using means of persuasion that point to the technical superiority of the new service in comparison with other providers. In the history of professionalization, however, the formation of clinical pharmacy represents a unique case: It is set within a wider profession that has no rival for drug-dispensing services. In contrast, when medicine professionalized at the end of the nineteenth century, claims to superiority were based on comparisons with the lesser trained homeopaths and folk healers. Eventually, around 1915, allopathic medicine began to receive state sanction through licensing. Clinical pharmacy cannot claim to be better than its competitors because, in fact, it has none. (True, many of the tasks it performs, and wants to perform, should be done by medicine to protect the health of patients, but often remain undone.) Therefore, positioning in the marketplace, a concrete way of advancing the sales of a product, is a difficult concept to apply to clinical pharmacy, since it is an altogether new service. Without an ill-trained, somewhat shabby competitor to hold up as a poor example as it calls for increasing professionalization, the clinically oriented segment of pharmacy has a difficult time drawing attention to itself. And it does not want to disaffect other pharmacists by offering them as the bad example.

Clearly, the clinical pharmacist, despite wishing to transform the profession, is a marginal figure in what has been called a marginal profession (McCormack 1956). Feelings of marginality are experienced by clinical pharmacists as they seek to lead pharmacy out of the wilderness, a form of leadership often associated in history with periods of social instability or rapid change (Lewin 1948).

Eliminating Restrictions on Practice

In order to stabilize and expand, clinical pharmacy must be sanctioned by state legislatures through amendments to licensing acts, approved by the courts, and funded by insurance plans or government programs. A stable and predictable market for its services cannot be established without these mechanisms permitting their delivery. Blue Cross and other health insurance underwriters do not prohibit reimbursement for clinical pharmacy services provided in hospitals. Reimbursement depends on the acceptance and approval of clinical services by administrative and medical staffs at each hospital. The market for clinical services, then, is not the third-party payer but the key medical personnel, who must regard the use of clinical pharmacy as necessary to good patient care. As a result of this decentralized arrangement, every pharmacist must be a lobbyist, for every hospital is a potential market. Consequently, certain strategies are ruled out, such as a concentrated and well-targeted lobbying campaign at Blue Cross headquarters or the federal Health Care Finance Administration. In this highly uncertain situation brought about by decentralization of the market, clinical pharmacists must develop and use skills in project preparation, cost-benefit analysis, and documentation of program effectiveness.

Equally important are the legal rights and responsibilities of clinical pharmacists. Some discussions of this issue imply that hospital pharmacists have a duty not only to prevent errors in filling prescriptions but also to guard against irrational drug therapy by physicians as well (Steves and Forrest 1969). In negligence cases, the courts have expected institutional pharmacists to exercise a high level of "due care," holding to a different standard of accountability than in cases involving community pharmacists (Fink 1980).

The clinical picture is even more complicated because it includes various activities such as drug history taking, maintaining patient medication profiles, drug monitoring, drug administration, drug prescribing, and patient consultation. The law is not completely clear on all aspects of clinical pharmacy practice, but DeMarco (1973, 549) has advised pharmacists to expand their services but proceed cautiously with clinical functions.

Upgrading of Responsibilities

The early rationale for expanding the functions of the hospital pharmacist was based on legal and technical foundations. Professionally oriented hospital pharmacists constituted an elite group that recommended increased involvement of their profession in decisions related to drugs prescribed in hospitals. While some progressive hospitals included pharmacists on their standing pharmacy and drug therapeutics committees, the 1965 amendments to the Social Security Act, which established Medicare, made the hospitals of the United States sensitive to the need to promote rational drug therapy. Under the law, payment or reimbursement to hospitals would be made only for approved drugs and biologicals, either those found in standard compendia or designated by Pharmacy and Therapeutics (P and T) committees (Provost 1965, 549).

The mishandling of drugs and biologicals in hospitals also became an issue in the 1960s. Since 1956, the Joint Commission on Hospital Accreditation has required that hospitals employ staff pharmacists. Some hospital pharmacists began to notice that nurses were doing "extemporaneous compounding" of parenterals — fluids administered intravenously or intramuscularly — for administration to hospitalized patients. Provost (1966, 595), in an editorial in the *AJHP*, viewed control over the compounding of these drugs in the hospital as the proper function of the pharmacist; nurses were not deemed sufficiently educated or skillful to continue performing this task. Along with taking this editorial position on compounding, the *AJHP* published many articles on the subject, some of them including a great deal of technical information on the potential incompatibilities of parenteral products.

No satisfactory answer exists as to why this technical function of "extemporaneous compounding" was in the hands of nurses in the first place, unless it was a carryover from the days when hospitals did not employ pharmacists. Pharmacists who were hired by hospitals and then served on P and T committees probably discovered these activities when they reviewed formulary orders and stock. At the same time, medicine began increased usage of parenteral fluids and drug dosage forms, sharpening the awareness of physicians and pharmacists alike of the potential for incompatible drug combinations. University-based pharmacists were quick to raise questions concerning quality control when drugs were handled casually: "Is it not inherently more dangerous to administer drugs intravenously than to give them orally? Does not the necessity for aseptic manipulations make the compounding of intravenous preparations even more difficult?" (Heller 1961, 520).

On the heels of this concern, pharmacists employed in hospitals developed the idea, based somewhat on community pharmacy or prescribing for ambulatory patients, of the "unit dose." Holding close to the view that pharmacy knew best how to prepare and deliver a patient's medication, they rejected the practice of simply placing batches of commonly used medications at nursing stations. If a prescription was written for an individual, they argued, a qualified pharmacist should do *all* the preparation, not just dispense medication to an intermediary (i.e., a nurse). After individualized prescription filling took place, nurses could then give an accurate and safe dosage to a patient (Jeffrey 1967).

Remuneration for Upgraded Activities

One may ask, How will these additional services provided by pharmacists be paid for? It follows that "professional fees" for hospital pharmacists are needed. Thus, pharmacists in hospitals ought to be paid for the technical skills used, regardless of the cost of the medication (Whitney and others 1968). Or so the argument runs. Always seeking to distance themselves from the commodity handled, leaders in hospital pharmacy advocated a standardized fee. The fee concept was introduced by hospital pharmacists in an attempt to lead the entire profession down the road to professionalization (Provost 1971, 17). Writers acknowledged that federally financed health insurance could implement this concept nationally, drawing on experiences of health service systems that gave professional fees to pharmacists, such as the health plan in Great Britain (Francke 1966, 171).

A professional fee was considered the key to societal recognition of pharmacy as a learned profession. The fee would provide a certain mystique to what might be considered a routine and ordinary task and transaction:

> The professional fee system separates the pharmacist from the role of the merchant and permits him to emphasize his professional role. A prescription is not an ordinary article of trade; it is an item whose distribution is limited by law to professional personnel (Francke 1966, 171).

What remained unrecognized was that the professional service rendered by the pharmacist, clinical or not, was directly tied to medication for sick people, even when distinct from the market value of the commodity. Still, the fee concept was looked on sympathetically by experts in hospital finance, now anxious to present a complete and detailed record of actual expenditures for services rendered to third party payers such as Blue Cross and Medicare. These new methods of accounting in the voluntary or nonprofit sector helped provide hospital pharmacy with a market for its service concept.

The change in hospital organization and financing brought about by third-party reimbursement systems was paralleled by the challenge of automation. Technology had already eliminated compounding and now threatened to reduce dispensing functions as well. Hospital pharmacy leaders saw this as an opportunity to perform clinical activities and thereby "attain new status." "Only the pharmacist by acting now can guarantee . . . he will free himself of routine, nonprofessional tasks and expand his role as a medication expert and drug therapy advisor" (Provost 1969, 199).

Much of the emphasis in hospital pharmacy in the late 1960s was on making drug therapy more rational. As a consultant to physicians, the hospital pharmacist would not only advise but review the way that prescribing was performed, and whether this task was done in the interest of the patient's health. Clinical leadership audaciously defined prescribing as a privilege, not a right, and one which would have to be constantly reviewed in order to be renewed (Provost 1970, 637). Somewhat later, the leadership suggested a more patient-oriented approach, coming up with the concept of clinical pharmacy, with the professional seizing the opportunity to offer these services. The new label only represented one step toward total reorganization (Provost 1971, 17). By the end of the 1970s, a national survey found that more than 60 percent of acute-care hospitals had partial or complete unit-dosage systems, and more than two-thirds had implemented at least a partial admixture (parenteral) system (Stolar 1979). Still at issue was the matter of professional fees and whether third-party payers would reimburse hospitals for clinical services to inpatients.

Aggressive Marketing of Services

Getting the hospital administrator to seek reimbursement for services was seen by editorial writers as the job of the pharmacists. Further, the American Society of Hospital Pharmacy (Reports 1981, 386) put forth detailed guidelines for its clinically oriented members to use to develop "acceptance and endorsement of the service by the involved administrative and medical staffs." The clinical movement members were directed "to channel their evangelism through the hospital department already in place for providing pharmaceutical services" (Zellmer 1981, 177). Pharmacists had been urged for a decade to leave the confines of the pharmacy and join other professions in planning the care of patients (Greiner 1972). But resistance to upgrading sometimes came from within pharmacy. Conversion activities were required.

> If any leader of such a department needs conversion, start there. If the department leaders are convinced, help them build the best clinical services feasible today. Then work with them and other colleagues in planning a strategy for redefining the hospital pharmacy as a clinical department of drug experts. (Zellmer 1981, 177)

Finding markets for clinical services means removing the fetters from pharmacy as well as convincing key people in hospital administration. Role expansion has to take place in order to establish a clinical profession amid a traditional dispensing practice; it also has to move into areas that were previously left undone or were based on the employment of a different labor supply. The nursing shortage of the 1980s was a recognized opportunity for pharmacy to demonstrate how clinical services could show substantial savings in nursing time. It was reasoned that some vacant nursing positions could be converted to the new role of medication administration technician — a new subprofessional who would prepare and give patients their unit dosage, and who would work under the direct supervision of the hospital pharmacy (Talley 1981, 45). The use of technicians hardly makes a field clinical, but supervising subprofessionals is status enhancing, being based on bureaucratic line authority. Such efforts at role expansion increase the number of role partners with which the incumbent interacts as a superior and as a peer with others who supervise. In a labor-intensive industry such as health care, people in middle management who are responsible for the personnel budget of a unit and employee relations (the terms of which are often dictated by union–management contract) get listened to by administrators. Moreover, under legal mandates for cost containment imposed by state and federal statutes, hospital pharmacy innovations that involve new appointments will hardly be entertained by administrators unless they are matched by employee reductions in other departments. Finally, cost-containing innovations in pharmacy now are used to market clinical services (Miyagawa and Rivera 1986).

Innovative Projects

In order to stimulate the public to demand the services they provide, clinically oriented pharmacists sought to make contact with patients through the development of innovative projects. The strategy was to find clinical problems that pharmacists could help solve. For years, physicians have complained that their therapies do not work because of patient noncompliance, and so a prospective market for patient services was readily identified. A second major problem, one brought on by therapy, was adverse drug reactions, one of the leading causes of hospitalization in the United States.

Adequate communication is central to helping maintain patient compliance and preventing adverse drug reactions. In the 1970s, the idea was introduced of a clinical pharmacist who receives information as well as uses knowledge to make an assessment to help solve or prevent other people's problems.

> A patient's pharmacist is familiar with the patient's medical and social history and his present health problems, and ensures that the patient's drug therapy is appropriate at all times. His knowledge-base includes an understanding of the clinical use and actions of drugs, pharmacokinetics, optimum clinical response, expected from drug therapy, monitoring and evaluating clinical response and communication skills for medication counseling. (Brands 1979, 312).

That pharmacists would give drug information was an unquestioned task advocated by clinical pharmacy's founders. Now the pharmacist would work for the patient, and he was instructed to acquire communication skills in order to elicit a complete medication history (Covington and Pfieffer 1972). Communication skills, by the nature of the extended relationship with patients, would be affective as well as cognitive. A more than fleeting relationship was to be established with the patient.

With the dreams of being the patient's pharmacist came new responsibilities. As a result of the extended contact, the process of death and dying was something that the pharmacist would now be required to see a patient through. Pharmacists always knew from the medication prescription they filled whether a patient (or customer) was terminally ill. Now they would be obligated to deal with this knowledge. Ongoing contact offered a new challenge to the pharmacist's communication skills. When a patient and family went through grief and bereavement, the structured relationship would include emotional as well as physical components. The stages of death and dying were made accessible to interested and involved pharmacists through articles customized to their new responsibilities (Wagner and Goldstein 1977).

Less dramatic, but equally demanding, would be the ongoing contact between the clinical pharmacist and the chronically ill. Here the case for involvement by clinical pharmacists could be made in a concrete way, since patients with asymptomatic diseases (e.g. hypertension) often have poor compliance records (Reinders, Rush, Baumgartner, and Graham 1975). Compliance among the chronically ill is not just an American medical problem; discussions of the ways to improve it are published in the pharmacy journals of other countries. (See Schrey and Ledwoch 1978; Ledwoch and others, 1978.)

Rather than integrate services to promote compliance among patients with prescription regimens, administrators have allowed pharmacists to establish clinics on an experimental basis. Physicians refer patients who are not complying with their medication regimens to the pharmacy. Using interviewing techniques, the clinician determines the reasons for noncompliance and attempts to alter behavior through verbal encouragement, special packaging (unit dosage), and medication calendars (Schneider and Cable 1978). While many of the efforts to induce greater patient compliance described in pharmacy journals have been self-proclaimed pilot programs to encourage others to test the clinical waters, some efforts have also been reported in medical publications (McKenny, Slining, Henderson, Davins, and Boor 1973).

Service for chronic care provided by the clinical pharmacist begin at discharge. Cancer patients, for example, receive brief monographs describing the nature and effects of the chemotherapeutic drugs included in their treatment (Stephens and McKinley 1976). Similar techniques have been employed with coronary care patients (Jinks 1974).

Specific skills in administering medication are also taught by pharmacists in home-care programs, a strategy being increasingly employed by hospital administrations through specific medical departments to reduce the need for lengthy hospitalization (Birenbaum 1981). These home-care programs have employed pharmacists to train patients to self-administer total parenteral nutrition solutions at home (Ivey, Riella, Mueller, and Scribner 1975).

American medicine has been criticized for failing to reach the poor and minority populations. Like other health-care professions, pharmacy has been involved in projects to compensate for the lack of medical services, reaching out to underserved populations such as rural Native Americans (Johnson and Tuchier 1975), the people of the hills and hollows of Appalachia (Baumgartner, Land, and Hauser 1972), and the inner-city minority poor (Mehl and Kissner 1972).

Less needy populations have been served in pilot programs. Adopting the protocol technique used in directing the physician assistant or nurse practitioner, pharmacists have managed specific disease populations of ambulatory patients receiving chronic drug therapy. In one project, protocols were established by agreement between pharmacists and physicians, thereby standardizing the questions asked and procedures undertaken in monitoring patients maintained on drugs: "In this system, the pharmacist interviews the patient, orders appropriate laboratory tests, evaluates the data and makes the decision regarding refill of medications. It is concluded that the clinically trained pharmacist can provide maintenance drug care" (Anderson and Taryle 1974, 255). The authors suggest that this clinical role cannot be performed simultaneously with the drug distribution function, and, two different types of pharmacy practitioners are therefore required.

Reviewing drug therapy for patients maintained on medication has become extremely important to avoid over- or-under-medication. One of the prime areas for acceptance of the services of clinical pharmacy has been through the performance of this function in skilled nursing facilities. In contrast to hospitals and ambulatory-care facilities, nursing homes have been less restrained in accepting clinical pharmacists. The great reliance on drug therapy, coupled with regulations requiring drug monitoring by the pharmacist, has led to the establishment of clinical practices in the service of the infirm elderly (Kidder 1977). General concern with adverse drug interactions for elderly patients is also noted, and the nursing home is one place to guard against this negative result of therapeutic intervention (Lipton and Lee 1988).

In one systematic study of drug regimens used in ten skilled nursing facilities, reviews indicated potential or real problems in 7.1 percent of 13,081 medical charts. The major sources of irrational therapy were prescribing with no documented indication of the need for medication or a lack of objective data for monitoring drug therapy effectiveness (Witte and others 1980). Over a four-year period, careful review of patient medication profiles by the pharmacist at a specific project at one skilled nursing facility led to a reduction of the average number of medications per patient from 7.7 to 6.1 (Rawlings and Fisk 1975).

Where long-term drug monitoring has been employed by health-care personnel, both acute and chronically ill patients have shown improvements and have suffered from fewer side effects from medications. In seeking to expand the clinical functions of pharmacy, programs have been established for previously hospitalized psychiatric patients in community settings. With the introduction of neuroleptic drugs, used to stabilize acutely psychotic patients, the pharmacist has been utilized to review the clinical responses of patients under medication (Evans and others 1976). In one community-care program for formerly hospitalized psychiatric patients, pharmacists and nurses decided whether to continue present drug therapy or initiate altered drug therapy (Ivey 1973). In another program,

> The pharmacist assesses stability of previously stabilized patients and may either refer a patient to the psychiatrist or work with the patient personally. If judged stable, the patient may be continued on the previous drug regimen. However, if the patient is mildly unstable or experiencing drug side effects, the pharmacist may alter dosage(s) or schedule(s), discontinue drug(s) and/or add drug(s). (Coleman, Evans, and Rosenbluth 1973, 1144)

All these roles are performed under a physician's standing orders. The kind of clinical work described above indicates that in this particular program, pharmacists were granted a great deal of responsibility and autonomy, similar to the way in which nurse practitioners and physician assistants were utilized in various health-care settings (see Chapter 4). Unlike the physician extenders, however, the clinical pharmacist often goes unnoticed by the public or is seen as simply a vendor of drugs, one unconcerned with the patient's health or the nation's capacity to pay for drug therapy.

The Dialectics of Professional Development

The practice of untraditional forms of pharmacy poses a dilemma within the profession as well as in the larger arena of health care. A pharmacist may be seen as a turncoat or as someone moving outside the profession when he performs clinical functions. The more different the clinical part of pharmacy becomes, as it develops, from the role of the traditional pharmacist, the more difficult it will be for the clinically oriented to remain within the field of pharmacy. Although there may be room for both traditional and untraditional pharmacists in the health-care field, clinical pharmacists are concerned about the image of their profession, hoping that the public and significant groups within the health-care field judge them by their contributions rather than outmoded expectations.

Clinical pharmacists are reformers who want to transform pharmacy into a profession that helps people solve their problems. An occupation that expands activities in this direction tries to apply knowledge in a specific domain, one in which it determines the nature of the service to be delivered and in which it can be clearly identified as expert.

The first tentative steps toward the development of a clear identification as an expert involve finding a problem area in which intervention is necessary and letting significant others know that your profession can contribute to preventing, containing, or solving that problem. By emphasizing problem identification, the clinical pharmacist shifts involvement from merely applying knowledge of medication formulation, called forth at the request of the physician, to communication of what the practitioners know about medications, their uses and interactions. The idea of pharmacists as drug-information experts, then, whether in the hospital or the community, puts them in a different social category and produces a different relationship with physicians, nurses, and even patients.

The new role of drug-information expert encourages pharmacists to act differently from traditional pharmacists, and they are treated differently. Their domain is not so directly tied to handling a commodity, something that has value in its own right and can be exchanged, but is founded on abstract knowledge. Further, since pharmacists are no longer acting only at the request of the physician, they are viewed as less supply bounded and therefore less passive. Organizationally, they are "staff" to decision makers; they have some influence, even to the extent of keeping physicians from making irreversible mistakes.

Whether branching out or breaking away, a crossroad that clinical pharmacy must come to someday, the movement has sought to organize a market for its services. In branching out throughout the 1970s, American clinical pharmacy sought structured contact with patients as well as advisory roles to healthcare personnel. Traditionally, community pharmacists have answered customer questions about over-the-counter medications, and how to administer prescriptions or packaged drugs; they have been asked to determine whether symptoms were serious enough to require a physician's examination. At the same time, advice and direction could come in health matters from anyone considered educated and in a position to make recommendations. When America was a less complex society than it is today, the local pharmacist was such an expert. The "docs" of the neighborhood drug stores always had some patient contact beyond the business transaction, although not everyone sought their advice and opinion. Often, customers filled a prescription on the run, using the most conveniently located shop or the one with late hours, and therefore did not ask questions or wait for unsolicited advice from the pharmacist. Undoubtedly, this relationship between pharmacist and consumer was a fleeting one. Although the advice at hand could be extremely helpful to the consumer, it was not an obligatory part of the relationship, but unexpected and requiring no recompense.

Not surprisingly, hospital-based pharmacists' contacts with patients were even less structured. In the public eye, hospital pharmacists hardly existed as a distinct group, separate from their community-based counterparts. Pharmacies were often located in hospital basements, along with the linen supplies. When pharmacists were noticed by the public (e.g., in contact with ambulatory-care patients), some confusion reigned. Hospital pharmacists recount anecdotes about patients who attempted to purchase over-the-counter drugs and sundries at their work stations or asked them for free calendars.

In stretching the boundaries of pharmacy, advocates of clinical pharmacy find themselves at odds with the traditional practitioner while making claims of providing substantial benefits through their intervention in patient care. The activities undertaken range from creating an awareness of services to conducting innovative projects in which pharmacists perform clinical services. The boundaries between traditional and clinical pharmacy are clear, if not well established. Advocates of clinical pharmacy seek to expand their cultural authority, primarily into domains considered important, but not claimed, by other professions. It remains to be seen whether the medical profession will encourage or discourage clinical pharmacy.

Two structural tendencies of contemporary American health care could heat up the boundary-work activities or introduce clinical pharmacy into practice more rapidly. First, the predicted oversupply of physicians may lead some doctors to adopt the procedures advocated by clinical pharmacists as part of their medical practice, leading to a new service for which remuneration can be requested. Second, as the rules for receiving remuneration in prospective payment systems become more standardized, the discretion in treatment exercised by physicians will be limited. The arguments and demonstrations engaged in by clinical pharmacists, which seek to convince the skeptical that hospitalization can be reduced through their efforts, may receive more attention by hospital administrators and physicians. In either case, a market for the services will be created, regardless of who delivers them.

References

Anderson, P.O., and D.A. Taryle. 1974. "Pharmacist management of ambulatory patients using formalized standards of care." *American Journal of Hospital Pharmacy* 31: 254–257.

Baumgartner, R.P., Jr., M.J. Land, and L.D. Hauser. 1972. "Rural health care – opportunity for innovative pharmacy service." *American Journal of Hospital Pharmacy* 29: 394–400.

Becker, M.H. 1985. "Patient adherence to prescribed therapies." *Medical Care* 23: 539–555.

Brands, A.J. 1979. "The patient's pharmacist." *American Journal of Hospital Pharmacy* 36: 311–315.

Broadhead, R.S., and N.J. Facchinetti. 1985. "Drug iatrogenesis and clinical pharmacy: The mutual fate of a social problem and a professional movement." *Social Problems* 35: 425–436.

Carter, W.B., T.S. Inui, W.A. Kukull, and, V.H. Haigh. 1982. "Outcome-based doctor-patient interaction analysis.II. Identifying effective provider and patient behavior."Medical Care: 20: 550.

Coleman, J.H., 3rd, R.L. Evans, and S.A. Rosenbluth. 1973. "Extended clinical roles for the pharmacist in psychiatric care." *American Journal of Hospital Pharmacy* 30: 1143–1146.

Covington, R.R., and F.G. Pfeiffer. 1972. "The pharmacist-acquired medication history." *American Journal of Hospital Pharmacy* 29: 692–696.

DeMarco, C.T. 1973. "The legal basis for clinical pharmacy practice." *American Journal of Hospital Pharmacy* 30: 1067–1071.

Evans, R.L., R.F. Kirk, P.W. Walker, S.A. Rosenbluth, and J. McDonald. 1976. "Medication maintenance of mentally ill patients by a pharmacist in a community setting." *American Journal of Hospital Pharmacy* 33: 635–638.

Fink, J.L. III. 1980. "Legal standard of due care for pharmacists in institutional practice." *American Journal of Hospital Pharmacy* 37: 1546–1549.

Fletcher C. 1978. "Listening and talking to patients I: The problem. II: The clinical interview. III: The exposition. IV: Some special problems." *British Medical Journal* 281: 845, 931, 994, 1056.

Francke, D.E. 1966. "Professional fees for pharmaceutical service." *American Journal of Hospital Pharmacy* 23: 171.

Gieryn, T.F. 1983. "Boundary-work and the demarcation of science from nonscience: Strains and interests in professional ideologies of scientists." *American Sociological Review* 48: 781–795.

Grauer, D.W. 1983. "Marketing concepts for pharmaceutical service development." *American Journal of Hospital Pharmacy* 38: 233–236.

Greiner, G.E. 1972. "The pharmacist's role in patient discharge planning." *American Journal of Hospital Pharmacy* 29: 72–76.

Hartoum, H.T., C. Catizone, R.A. Hutchinson, and A. Purohit. 1986. "An eleven year review of the pharmacy literature: Documentation of the value and acceptance of clinical pharmacy." *Drug Intelligence and Clinical Pharmacy* 20 (January): 33–48.

Haynes, R.B., D.W. Taylor, and D.L. Sackett, eds. 1979. *Compliance in Health Care.* Baltimore: Johns Hopkins University Press.

Heller, W.M. 1961. "Should the pharmacist assume additional responsibilities for medication preparation?" *American Journal of Hospital Pharmacy* 18: 520.

Ivey, M.F., M. Riella, W. Mueller, and B. Scribner. 1975. "Long- term parenteral nutrition in the home." *American Journal of Hospital Pharmacy* 32: 1032–1036.

Ivey, M.F. 1973. "The pharmacist in the care of ambulatory mental health patients." *American Journal of Hospital Pharmacy* 300: 599–602.

Jeffrey, L.P. 1967. "Professional considerations in drug distribution systems." *American Journal of Hospital Pharmacy* 24: 60–62.

Jinks, M. 1974. "The hospital pharmacist in an interdisciplinary inpatient teaching program." *American Journal of Hospital Pharmacy* 31: 569–573.

Johnson, R.E., and R.J. Tuchier. 1975. "Role of the pharmacist in primary health care." *American Journal of Hospital Pharmacy* 32: 162–164.

Keefer, C.S. 1966. "A physician looks at drug information." *American Journal of Hospital Pharmacy* 23: 55–59.

Kidder, S.W. 1977. "Skilled nursing facilities—a clinical opportunity for pharmacists." *American Journal of Hospital Pharmacy* 34: 751–753.

Larson, M.S. 1977. *The Rise of Professionalism: A Sociological Analysis.* Berkeley: University of California Press.

Ledwoch, W., and others. 1978. "Patient compliance—underestimated problem?" *Pharmazeutische Zeitung* 123 (October 12): 1774-1779.

Lewin, K. 1948. *Resolving Social Conflicts, Part III.* New York: Harper & Row.

Lipton, Helene L., and Philip R. Lee. 1988. *Drugs and the Elderly: Clinical, Social and Policy Perspectives.* Stanford: Stanford University Press.

Marston, M.V. 1977. "Nursing management of compliance with medical regimens." In *Medication Compliance: A Behavioral Management Approach,* edited by I. Barofsky, 139-164. Thorofare, N.J.: Charles B. Slack.

McCormack, T.H. 1956. "The druggist's dilemma: Problems of a marginal occupation." *American Journal of Sociology* 61: 308–315.

McKenny, J.M., J.M. Slining, H.R. Henderson, D. Davins, and M. Boor. 1973. "The effect of clinical pharmacy services on patients with essential hypertension." *Circulation* 48: 1104-1111.

Mehl, B., and E.A. Kissner. 1972. "Ambulatory pharmaceutical services in a changing urban community." *American Journal of Hospital Pharmacy* 29: 407–410.

Miyagawa, C.I., and J.O. Rivera. 1986. "Effect of pharmacist interventions on drug therapy costs in a surgical intensive- care unit." *American Journal of Hospital Pharmacy* 43 (December): 3008–3013.

Nardone, D.A., J.B. Reuler, and D.E. Girard. 1980. "Teaching history-taking: where are we?" *Yale Journal of Biological Medicine* 53: 233.

Pendleton, D.A. 1983. "Doctor–patient communication. A review." In *Doctor-Patient Communication,* edited by D. Pendleton and J. Halster. London: Academic.

Pendleton, D.A., H. Brouwer, and J. Jaspars. 1983. "Communications difficulties: the doctor's perspective." *Journal of Language and Social Psychology* 2: 17.

Platt, F.W. 1981. "Research in medical interviewing." *Annals of Internal Medicine* 94: 405.

Platt, F.W., and J.C. McMath. 1979. "Clinical hypocompetence: the interview." *Annals of Internal Medicine* 91: 898.

Provost, G.P. 1965. "Hospital pharmacy under Medicare." *American Journal of Hospital Pharmacy* 22: 549.

_____. 1966. "Prescription compounding by nurses in hospitals." *American Journal of Hospital Pharmacy* 23: 595.

_____. 1969. "The challenge of automation." *American Journal of Hospital Pharmacy* 26: 199.

_____. 1970. "Drug prescribing as a privilege." *American Journal of Hospital Pharmacy* 27: 637.

_____. 1971. "Clinical pharmacy and hospital pharmacy." *American Journal of Hospital Pharmacy* 28: 17.

Rawlings, J.L., and P.A. Fisk. 1975. "Pharmaceutical services for skilled nursing facilities in compliance with federal regulations." *American Journal of Hospital Pharmacy* 32: 905–908.

Reinders, T.P., D.R. Rush, P. Baumgartner Jr., and A.W.Graham. 1975. "Pharmacist's role in management of hypertensive patients in an ambulatory care clinic." *American Journal of Hospital Pharmacy* 32: 590.

Reiser, D.E., and A.D. Schroder. 1980. *Patient Interviewing: The Human Dimension.* Baltimore: Williams and Wilkins.

Reports, *AJHP.* 1981. "ASHP guidelines for implementing and obtaining reimbursement for clinical pharmaceutical services." *American Journal of Hospital Pharmacy* 38: 386.

Schneider, P., and G. Cable. 1978. "Compliance clinic: An opportunity for an expanded practice role for pharmacists." *American Journal of Hospital Pharmacy* 35: 288–295.

Schrey, A., and W. Ledwoch. 1978. "Role of the pharmacist in improving patient compliance." *Deutche Apotheker-Zeitung* 118 (May 18): 724–727.

Schwartz, M.A. 1976. "The role of the pharmacist in the patient-health team relationship." In *Patient Compliance*, edited by I. Barofsky, 83-95. Mount Kisco, NY: Future Publishing

Sharpe, T.R. 1977. "The pharmacist's potential role is a factor in increasing compliance." *In Medication Compliance: A Behavioral Management Approach* edited by I. Barofsky, 113–138. Thorofare, NJ: Charles B. Slack.

Starr, P. 1982. *The Social Transformation of American Medicine: The Rise of a Sovereign Profession and the Making of a Vast Industry.* New York: Basic Books.

Steeves, R.F., and T.P. Forrest. 1969. "Legal responsibility of the hospital pharmacist for rational drug therapy." *American Journal of Hospital Pharmacy* 26: 404–407.

Stephens, S.P., and J.D. McKinley Jr. 1976. "Pharmaceutical services for the cancer patient." *American Journal of Hospital Pharmacy* 33: 1141-1145.

Stolar, M.H. 1979. "National survey of hospital pharmaceutical services— 1978." *American Journal of Hospital Pharmacy* 36: 316-325.

Talley, C.R. 1981. "Aspirin for the nursing shortage headache: Upgrade pharmaceutical services." *American Journal of Hospital Pharmacy* 38: 45.

Wagner, J., and E. Goldstein. 1977. "Pharmacist's role in loss and grief." *American Journal of Hospital Pharmacy* 34. 490–492.

Whitney, H.A.K., Jr., D.C. McLeod, and R.W. Richards. 1968. "A new definition of the pharmacist's fee." *American Journal of Hospital Pharmacy* 25: 691-693.

Witte, K.W., N.H. Leeds, D.S. Pathak, K.D. Campagna, D.P. West, and A.L. Spunt. 1980. "Drug regimen review in skilled nursing facilities by consulting clinical pharmacists." *American Journal of Hospital Pharmacy* 37: 820–824.

Zellmer, W.A. 1981. "Integrated or independent clinical services?" *American Journal of Hospital Pharmacy* 38: 17.

7 **The Expansion of Pharmacy and the Shortfall in Clinical Positions: Discontinuities Between Production and Distribution**

Clinical pharmacy is a product of the social conditions of its time. It follows the paths laid down by dominant professions. Professions in America, especially dominant ones, go through cycles of corruption and reform, with ethically suspect behavior taking place mainly in times of economic expansion, followed by efforts at ethical renewal during times when the market for services diminishes. They may set the pattern for all kinds of reforms, even when professional misconduct is not at issue.

Pharmacy is no exception to this pattern because the reformers certainly were anticipating a shrinking market for traditional pharmacy services, given the technological and financial changes in the drug industry and health-care service-delivery system. In addition to these threats to pharmacists, there are now concerns about a loss of status directly resulting from the extensive development of chain stores and mail-order distributors that are not owned by pharmacists. This double threat of loss or displacement — both power and status — makes the collective mobility project of reformers in pharmacy more complex than anticipated and leads to negative fallout from newly educated clinical pharmacists who wait in the wings to take on new responsibilities.

Reforms in pharmacy education, necessary to sustain the collective mobility project, are going through without much opposition in colleges of pharmacy. Yet there are many barriers to clinical practice, some of them put there to make sure that only pharmacists could do certain tasks in hospitals, thereby creating

140

stable sources of income as well as numerous staff positions. Now, these legal protections, found in state codes concerning health institutions and their staffing, are fetters on professional growth and increased income.

Another roadblock in the way of the clinical pharmacy movement is the trend in occupational development in community pharmacy. The growth of chain-store pharmacies has increased the number of jobs available in those locations, at salaries that are usually higher than those found in hospitals, where clinical pharmacy is more likely to be practiced. According to 1987 figures, 42.4 percent of all the college of pharmacy graduates were hired by chain pharmacies (American Association of Colleges of Pharmacy 1987). Opportunities to practice clinical pharmacy are limited in these settings. The structure and culture of pharmacy are moving in opposite directions.

At the end of the 1980s, chain or discount pharmacies are continuing to expand and are driving owner/operator pharmacies out of business. Heavily capitalized, these chains fill prescriptions for a large volume trade, leaving little time for pharmacists to advise the public on the proper use of medications. Despite the better opportunities for employment and excellent starting salaries, I expect that dissatisfaction with work is strongest among pharmacists employed in these businesses because they have a heavy workload and little opportunity to own a pharmacy, alone or in partnership, because of heavily capitalization requirements. In many ways, the chain-store pharmacist is the forgotten professional in the effort to create a clinical profession.

To what extent does identification with the aspirations of the profession remain? Kronus (1976) found hospital pharmacists identified with the medical profession; independent pharmacy owners viewed themselves as linked to their fellow owner/operators of community pharmacies; and chain-store pharmacists identified with consumers. This last form of identification deserves comment because of its unusual nature. It is plausible that those in positions of little power identify with another powerless group, the consumers. Moreover, this kind of response represents a situation of normative ambiguity or marginality in a rapidly changing occupational world.

Professional developments can move simultaneously in opposite directions. It would appear that a dual process of reprofessionalization and deprofessionalization is occurring in pharmacy. Within the heavily capitalized chain store, pharmacists distribute manufactured products as wage workers. Thus, labor has been heavily rationalized, that is, under the control of capital, following the model outline by Marx in 1857.

> The accumulation of knowledge and of skill, of the general productive forces of the social brain, is thus absorbed into capital, as opposed to labour, and hence appears as an attribute of capital, and more specifically of *fixed capital*, in so far as it enters into the production process as a means of production proper. (Marx 1978, 280; italics in original)

In contrast, when clinical pharmacists are able to practice, and thereby able to renew their human capital, they are making profits beyond what they need to survive and getting more skilled at what they do. In essence, the professional resists the processes of rationality induced by fixed capital. According to Larson (1977), the basis of the power and status of the professional is that their knowledge and skill cannot be divorced from their labor.

> The possessions appropriated by the professional consist, typically, of practical and theoretical knowledge, under the form of a special *competence*. This form of property has two distinctive character-istics: on the one hand, it is inseparable from mind and self; on the other, it constitutes a resource that cannot be depleted. (Larson 1977, 222; italics in original)

The younger and better-educated pharmacists are prepared to do clinical work, that, by and large, is not available in suffi-cient quantities to accommodate all those interested in it. Educational reforms are far ahead of practice opportunities. And simply advocating an upgrading of all pharmacy education to the doctoral level, making the Pharm.D. degree the entry re-quirement into the profession for all, will not place all the graduates into clinical positions.

It is possible to train pharmacy technicians and delegate most routine tasks to them in order to free the pharmacist to do clinical work. But, the earlier lobbying efforts by state pharmacy societies would have to be undone so that pharmacists could be freed from the exclusive responsibilities for preparing medication, permitting them to delegate tasks. Observers complain that the system created is irrational, since "pharmacy practice regulations in most states *require* that pharmacists perform various technical and manipulative functions which could easily be performed by others" (Ray 1977, 579; italics in original).

Reforms in Education and Opportunities to Practice Clinical Pharmacy

Encouraged by the widely acclaimed Millis Report on the need for reform in pharmacy education, many colleges of pharmacy revised their curriculum to reflect a new emphasis on the drug advisory activities of pharmacists in hospitals and in the community. By the middle of the 1970s, colleges of pharmacy had begun to stress that their graduates would be performing clinical functions in relation to patients and physicians, since pharmacists were experts in drug information. In essence, function would follow education reform.

Newly educated pharmacists have been employed in various settings for a number of years. Currently, however, clinical practice in pharmacy takes place in relatively few hospitals, mainly those with a tradition for innovative health care services. Conducted in 1978, a national sample survey of pharmaceutical services at 815 acute-care hospitals suggested that clinical services are most cost effective at large hospitals (Stolar 1979). Based on projections from the sample, at that time only 150 hospital pharmacies in the United States provided a comprehensive clinical service program. Most of these hospitals had over 400 beds and were located in New England or on the Pacific Coast. (Although such information was not provided, it is likely that these hospitals are affiliated with medical and pharmacy schools.)

In a survey of midwestern hospitals, those who got to practice clinical pharmacy were more satisfied with their work than staff pharmacists (Johnson, Hammel, and Heinen 1977, 241). In another study in the Midwest, when institutional and community pharmacists were compared, no differences in satisfaction were found. One exception to this overall result was that practitioners in ethical pharmacies — where no sundries are sold — reported higher levels of satisfaction than pharmacists in other settings (Curtis, Hammel, and Johnson 1978, 1516). Opportunities to engage in clinical practice, such as consulting with patients and physicians, were found by Watkins and Norwood (1978) in their study of consulting behavior of pharmacists located in service-oriented and discount pharmacies. Pharmacists practicing in service-oriented locations were more likely to advise physicians about potential problems than their equally knowledgeable counterparts in the chain stores.

It is important to report on discontinuities between education and practice in order to determine not only what settings encourage the practice of clinical pharmacy but what strategies are employed by newly educated pharmacists to accomplish this objective. Moreover, recent graduates constitute an important source of information because they are less likely to have become cynical about professionalism than more veteran pharmacists.

In a study of graduates of two schools of pharmacy in New York City, my colleagues and I found that 54 percent of the sample were disappointed with their work because their "knowledge goes far beyond filling prescriptions." Moreover, of the 37 percent of respondents who were satisfied with their current work situation, half claimed that their work was clinical in nature. Thus, no more than 19 percent of this sample of recent graduates of colleges of pharmacy, which now follow a revised curriculum, saw themselves as performing clinical roles (Birenbaum, Bologh, and Lesieur 1987, 292).

In this study, we examined perceptions and expectations about work, differences in consulting practices, relationships between practice and attitudes, and the presence of an identifiable general value orientation (which could account for specific perceptions and attitudes). Results indicated that hospital practice was more likely to be associated with clinical pharmacy, and clinical pharmacy practice was more likely to meet the expectations of recently graduated pharmacists. In addition, and surprisingly, 52 percent of the community-based pharmacists were engaged in patient counseling, compared with 39 percent of hospital-based pharmacists (Birenbaum, Bologh, and Lesieur, 1987).

Hospital pharmacy is the usual place where clinical pharmacy is practiced, but not every hospital pharmacist practices it. In fact, the lack of opportunities to engage in clinical practice may be more keenly felt by hospital pharmacists, who can observe their peers doing clinical work; community pharmacists, in contrast, not only do not see their differences but may well have access to compensatory responsibilities in management and marketing. Nevertheless, the most satisfied pharmacists were those who perceived their work as consultative in nature, not merely commercial or technical.

Recent graduates with a more clinical orientation are more likely to cite the business aspects of pharmacy as a problem of the profession, yet the relationship between the general value orientation of professionalism and the particular perception of problems is complex. Pharmacists in the community who are assertive professionally (i.e., insist on making time available to consult with patients) downgrade the difficulties that commercialism engenders. The presence of this group may be viewed as the result of competitive individualism rising above the structural constraints of business or may stem from a secure belief that there is professional group support behind them.

In the light of the limited opportunities to practice clinical pharmacy, it would be reasonable to suggest that pharmacists trained as clinicians cannot retain their clinical skills if they are not able to practice; nor can they remain motivated to work with patients. Failure to find avenues for advancement along clinical lines means that those with strong ambitions will seek managerial positions to advance their careers. Unlike medicine, where the skilled clinician receives many referrals and is able to advance in his practice, the pharmacist's career pattern resembles that found in nursing, where advancement means going into administration or teaching.

Advocates of clinical pharmacy recognize the dangers of trying to hold on to the new purpose of the profession when opportunities are lacking. At the same time, there is concern that the clinical movement is segmenting the profession: "With clinical pharmacy gaining acceptance, we must find a way to keep competent clinically oriented "staff" pharmacists—those who work primarily in patient care areas and who want to remain there—by giving them opportunity for advancement without isolating them from the mainstream" (Provost 1969, 565).

Reinventing Pharmacy Education and Educators

Using the methods of science to evaluate their impact on patients, clinical pharmacy pilot projects could affect patient behavior and health outcomes. The problem remains, however, to demonstrate that pharmacy education has changed radically, producing the capacity for widely found standard interventions that help patients.

A focus on producing a service makes it possible to show the advantages of clinical pharmacy. A focus on the *reproduction* of service providers—through selection and training—puts this newly acquired expertise solely in the hands of the profession as an occupational community. Something special is suggested in this step in production: The service provided is unique insofar as it is available only from these specifically identified practitioners (clinical pharmacists) and, equally important, the holders of the professional license or degree are relatively uniform in their abilities.

By taking command of the curriculum of colleges of pharmacy, advocates of reprofessionalization claim to possess a substantial body of technical and clinical knowledge that they can transmit to students through classroom and practical education. This transmission process can take place only in a sheltered environment (i.e., the university) where the discovery of new knowledge is approved and where standardized information can be imparted to novices. Placing education and training in the university and the hospital is a way of emulating the other learned professions; it is also quite clearly a way of identifying with the entire health-care endeavor.

A primary consideration in the production of producers is the development of a faculty competent to teach at the university level. In addition, supervised clinical settings, such as hospital internships, are required. Finally, to be truly clinical, the curriculum needs to incorporate the behavioral and social sciences as well as the physical and biological sciences.

The production of an experienced faculty requires access to clinical practice settings which pharmacists have traditionally been denied. It is useful to consider the problems facing the faculties of colleges of pharmacy from a structural perspective. First, how can they overcome the traditional separation of pharmacy faculties from hospitals and other medical settings so that they can gain the clinical experience necessary to guide their students? And, second, how will they acquire the knowledge and beliefs about patient behavior and attitudes that has to be imparted to students, when such matters are not defined as significant to the practice of pharmacy (e.g., illness behavior)? It is apparent that the pharmacy faculty must not only expand its roles but its role partners if it is to gain access and knowledge.

Breaking down traditional barriers to partnerships with physicians, hospital administrators, or even the social sciences will be difficult. Students in field placements may be more adept at understanding patients and their beliefs than the clinical pharmacy faculty. Such anomalous situations are likely to exist for a number of years. In regard to the social sciences, advocates of clinical pharmacy are likely to absorb the values and ideas of the social sciences and then reject the rights of these disciplines to contribute to pharmacy education. The only way this can be avoided is if more interdisciplinary education is available so that all students in the health sciences take courses together from social scientists concerned with patient-care issues.

The new education of the clinical pharmacist requires the creation of a curriculum to educate pharmacy technicians to take over dispensing functions. In upgrading pharmacy education, the market value of the newly trained professional is increased, even when no actual service has been provided. Since colleges of pharmacy have a monopoly on instructing pharmacists, and since pharmacy practice requires a degree, the profession can seek to increase its "professional exchange value" unilaterally (Larson 1977, 211). Without a monopoly on a task considered vital, internal consistency in education will not ensure the success of the profession's collective mobility project.

Much of the opportunity to practice clinical pharmacy will come from overcoming resistance from within the profession. In addition, physicians who occupy major decision-making positions in hospitals need to be convinced that clinical pharmacy is as important to health-care delivery as its advocates say it is.

Physician Response

A consistent finding in studies is that physicians hold negative attitudes toward clinical roles for pharmacists. Viewed mainly as technicians by physicians, pharmacists are considered the wrong professionals to make decisions concerning choice of drugs for patients (Ritchey and Raney 1981a; 1981b). Interestingly, these studies found physicians to have more favorable attitudes toward physician assistants, than pharmacists, when it came to monitoring drug therapy for patients with chronic diseases.

The legitimacy of expanding the pharmacist role was studied through a survey of nurses, pharmacists and physicians in California. In none of the samples was the return rate for the mailed questionnaire above 45 percent, and the response rate for a sample of 200 randomly selected Los Angeles physicians was a mere 31 percent. Adamcik and her colleagues (1986, 1193) found little support for both triage and general advisement activities performed by pharmacists in hospital settings. Even less support was evinced for pharmacists performing clinical activities in the community setting. In fact, the majority of physicians sampled (63 percent) did not consider pharmacists to be health-care professionals (Adamcik and others 1986, 1196). Physicians who had contact with clinical pharmacists were more likely than those who did not have contact to support role expansion for pharmacists in the community. These findings supported the view that clinical pharmacy, particularly in the

community, where the pharmacist cannot be monitored or controlled, is regarded by the organized profession of medicine as a
threat to its power. (In other words, a community pharmacist
who gives advice might be steering a patient away from a medical
consultation.) Medical authority in the area of prescribing and
how to take medications has been sovereign for a half a century.

The Material Foundation of the Physician's Authority

Physicians gained legal control over drug distribution in
the United States fifty years ago. In response to a large number
of deaths caused by using untested drugs, Congress in 1938 passed
laws designed to regulate the testing, marketing, and use of so-
called dangerous drugs; and physicians became responsible for
protecting the public from the misuse of these potent prescriptions. In essence, physicians were put in charge of drug safety;
very few effective drugs were available over-the-counter. The
doctor, in essence, became the patient's agent when prescribing
pharmaceutical products, guaranteeing the safety of the product to
be consumed. The new controls and safeguards made doctors the
gatekeepers who regulated the flow of pharmaceuticals in society.
In a sense, clinical pharmacy seeks to take over that role.

Legal authority produced a great material advantage for
doctors, an advantage ratified by the drug industry. Once access
to medication required prescriptions, doctors became very important figures for pharmaceutical houses since doctors triggered
the dispensing process. Only recently, with the widespread use
of generic drugs, are brand-name producers seeking to reach actual consumers and get them to influence a doctor's decision in
prescribing (Altman 1988). No wonder that drug producers developed close relationships with physicians in order to influence
their decisions in prescribing (Temin 1980, 88). A new alliance
was born, making manufacturers dependent on doctors for sales
and doctors reliant on advertisements and detail men of the industry for information and guidance as to what to prescribe and
who in the medical community was adopting which drug therapies
(Temin 1980, 118).

If the movement toward clinical pharmacy is to achieve legitimacy, medicine must be convinced that there is a need for involving pharmacists in rational drug therapy; to do this physicians must also change their customary practice of consultation on drugs. The acquisition of new responsibilities by pharmacists depends on whether medicine can be convinced that it should delegate legally mandated responsibilities to another health profession. Currently, some doctors in the United States are stocking and dispensing medications directly to patients, eliminating the need for the consumers to go to a pharmacy.

The information explosion in medicine and health care justifies some specialization in the area of drug information. In the doctor's world, observers point out that between 1978 and 1982, pharmaceutical companies have marketed 450 new drugs in the United States. Companies must rely on increasingly specialized representatives to spread the word among doctors on how the drugs should be used (Altman 1982, C3). Pharmacists as well as physicians have to know how drugs should be used in order to prevent medication errors and answer questions by consumers.

Pharmacists also occasionally inform physicians as to the availability of new medications. And sometimes, pharmacists are asked to inform *on* physicians, letting the drug manufacturer's division of marketing collect data on the prescribing habits of physicians whose patients frequent their pharmacies. Some pharmacists regard the divulgence of this information as unethical while others see it as simply a matter of public record (Altman 1982, C3).

For the industry, influencing a physician's choice of medication is a serious business. Manufacturers become desperate to maintain their market shares once they lose their sheltered-status; patents protect new products from competition for seventeen years and brand names for forty years. Sales have been helped along by the wide acceptance and use of medical intervention in health matters in our society. Every year, more and more people are seen by physicians in office visits. This increase in customary usage of services offered by doctors helps the pharmaceutical industry avoid the uncertainties found in other industries. Prescription drugs, unlike cars and candy bars, are not directly subject to market fluctuations; their consumption depends on prescribed necessary use, regardless of boom or recession. Physicians, then, have become key gatekeepers in the use of pharmaceuticals, and manufacturers have focused their attention on getting their message across to them. In the course of cultivating the profession of medicine, the industry has unwittingly helped make it a very powerful institution in American society.

The AMA played a key role in opening the gates to the manufacturers to reach their membership. Brand-name advertisements in the seventeen journals of the association have been one mechanism for reaching physicians, and helped fill the coffers of the AMA. Once considered unethical by the AMA, brand-name advertising became a way of generating income subsequently used in the service of the medical profession's powerful lobbying activities against various government-sponsored national health insurance programs. When seeking to gain societal recognition through state licensing, medical reformers of the Progressive era viewed advertizing in professional journals as undignified, commercial, and professionally compromising. This policy was altered in the late 1940s when President Truman first proffered a national health insurance act, and the AMA sought to develop a war chest to fight "socialized medicine."

The transfer of funds through advertising in the pages of medical journals was necessary because the industry needed to maintain a demand of great magnitude and constancy. The payments were no hardship when corporations realized the highest rates of return of any American industry: "The drug companies regularly show a return of about 18 percent, a figure two-thirds higher than the average rate of return for all manufacturing concerns in the decade 1960–1970" (Goddard 1981, 248).

The power of the industry lies in its resources and its capacity to get the professions dependent on it. Not only have manufacturers sought support from the AMA for antisubstitution laws for prescriptions written for brand-name products, but they have attempted to influence the profession of pharmacy as well. Using support from national pharmacy organizations, such as the American Pharmaceutical Association and the National Association of Boards of Pharmacy, the National Pharmaceutical

Council, a trade association, was formed by twelve companies in 1953 to pass antisubstitution legislation. The professional associations of pharmacy argued that concern for public safety required the use of brand names. In joining the trade association, pharmacy leaders rationalized their involvement as based on pure professionalism rather than pecuniary concerns. At the time of their involvement, retail pharmacy owners sought to prevent the substitution of generic drugs so that they could commercially stabilize their retail businesses. A law of this kind would buttress advancement toward the goal of having one price charged by all pharmacies. The independent pharmacies sought to eliminate volume purchasing and other marketing advantages held by chain-store and discount pharmacies. Professionalism and controlling competition, as is often the case, were mutually supportive goals (Facchinetti and Dickson 1982, 471). Trade associations even went so far as to seek legislation to prevent over-the-counter medications from being sold outside drug stores.

The industry was able to get legislative support for antisubstitution legislation by waging a campaign against a nonexistent public health problem. While the industry argued passionately that generic drugs were substandard, it offered no evidence to substantiate this claim. In fact, the opposite conclusion was drawn by those who bothered to check the data on quality of generic versus brand name drugs. Senator Estes Kefauver, a noted critic of big business, on following the hearings on the drug industry, inferred that generic substitution should be expanded rather than reduced, thereby passing on savings to consumers and third-party payers of prescription costs.

But manufacturers managed to carry the day with the help of the national pharmacy associations, which obligingly lent the industry a mantle of professional prestige. Legislative bodies in thirty-eight states were convinced that substitution should be restricted in prescription filling, even when physician judgment permitted it (Facchinetti and Dickson 1982, 473). The industry made the cost of entry for new manufacturers extremely high with this protective legislation (Perrow 1979, 214). The industry continued to teach physicians that effective drugs are associated only with trade names (Barnhart 1976, 116). The physicians obliged by prescribing them and demonstrating to the public that they knew how to control and use drugs safely.

Chemically, trade or brand-name drugs and the generics may differ slightly, but therapeutically they are the same. Physicians have not made efforts to challenge the industry's claim that brand names are more effective than generic drugs, despite the Food and Drug Administration testing of the two, which found no differences. Furthermore, some academic physicians, including the dean of the Harvard Medical School, have explicitly warned colleagues against the professionally dubious distinction they often make in their work between brand name and generic drugs (Barnhart 1976, 111–112).

Value-minded people, led by consumer activists, began to mount a campaign in the 1960s to rescind the antisubstitution laws. The idea of using generic drugs was a powerful one in the hands of a sophisticated backlash to manipulative advertising.

> Not being able to choose prescription drugs for themselves, they wanted to restrict the doctor's power to order expensive drugs for them when cheaper equivalents were available. To be sure, this would simply shift the decision to the pharmacist, not the consumer, but the opponents of the anti-substitution laws assumed that pharmacists were not as much the object of advertisements for brand name drugs and were more subject to legislative control. Over thirty states had repealed their anti-substitution laws by 1977. Two-thirds of these, however, did not give pharmacists license to substitute whenever they wished; they furnished either a list of substitutable drugs or a list of non-substitutable drugs to restrict their actions. (Temin 1980, 159)

The implications for clinical pharmacy are apparent. On the one hand, the revision of state laws permitting substitution of generic for brand-name products should create more professional responsibility for pharmacists when dispensing. On the other hand, as gatekeepers to medication, physicians are clearly reluctant to delegate responsibility in this area of providing treatment to those who are not under their direct supervision. With the cultural authority to design care systems, as well as to treat patients with drugs, strongly in the hands of physicians, there would seem to be a limit on the growth of clinical pharmacy in the current century.

Alternatively, if reimbursements are capped for services and comprehensive providers such as HMOs seek to prevent iatrogenic disorders, rehospitalization, and other drains on the resources of providers, then the innovative introduction of services by clinical pharmacists may be cost effective. At the same time, any rationing system called for will be based on designing comprehensive coverage, following existing utilization patterns, thereby discouraging innovations in service delivery. As in the past, and as it is theoretically predictable, the growth and development of professions are strongly influenced by state policy and requirements. In the next chapter, I examine where this movement and the physician extender movements are heading, and why.

References

Adamcik, Barbara A., and others. 1986. "New clinical roles for pharmacists: A study of role expansion." *Social Science and Medicine* 23: 1187-2000.

Altman, Lawrence. 1982. "The doctor's world: Is medicine helped by sales tactics of 'detailmen'?" *New York Times* (July 6) C3.

_____. 1988. "The doctor's world: New drug ads bear implications for physicians." *New York Times* (March 2) C2.

American Association of Colleges of Pharmacy. 1987. *Reports* 1986-7: 3.

Barnhart, Rick. 1976. "Getting a fix: The U.S. drug monopoly." In *Prognosis Negative: Crisis in the Health Care System*, edited by David Kotelchuch, 107-124. New York: Vintage.

Birenbaum, Arnold, Roslyn Bologh, and Henry Lesieur. 1987. "Reforms in pharmacy education and opportunity to practice clinical pharmacy." *Sociology of Health and Illness: a Journal of Medical Sociology* 9 (September): 286-301.

Curtis, F.R., R.J. Hammel, and C.A. Johnson. 1978. "Psychological strain and job dissatisfaction in pharmacy practice: Institutional vs. community practitioners." *American Journal of Hospital Pharmacy* 35 (December): 1516-1520.

Facchinetti, Neil J., and W. Michael Dickson. 1982. "Access to generic drugs in the 1950s: The politics of a social problem." *American Journal of Public Health* 72 (May): 468-475.

Goddard, James L. 1981. "The medical business." *The Sociology of Health and Illness: Critical Perspectives*, edited by Peter Conrad and Rochelle Kern, 247–254. New York: St. Martin's Press.

Johnson, C.A., R.S. Hammel, and J.S. Heinen. 1977. "Levels of satisfaction among hospital pharmacists." *American Journal of Hospital Pharmacy* 34 (March): 241–247.

Kronus, Carol L. 1976. "Occupational vs. organizational influences in reference group identification: The case of pharmacy." *Sociology of Work and Occupations* 3 (August): 303–331.

Larson, Margali Safatti. 1977. *The Rise of Professionalism: A Sociological Analysis*. Berkeley: University of California Press.

Marx, Karl. 1978. "The Grundrisse." In *The Marx-Engels Reader*, edited by Robert C. Tucker, 221–293. 2nd edition. New York: Norton.

Perrow, Charles. 1979. *Complex Organizations: A Critical Essay*. 2nd Ed. Glenview, Ill.: Scott, Foresman.

Provost, George P. 1969. "Removing the dead end in clinical pharmacy." *American Journal of Hospital Pharmacy* 26: 565.

Ray, Max. 1977. "In support of one degree for pharmacy." *American Journal of Hospital Pharmacy* 34: 579–580.

Ritchey, F.J., and M.R. Raney. 1981a. "Medical role-task boundary maintenance: Physicians' opinions of clinical pharmacy." *Medical Care* 19: 90.

_____. 1981b. "Effect of exposure on physicians' attitudes toward clinical pharmacists." *American Journal of Hospital Pharmacy* 38: 1459.

Stolar, Michael H. 1979. "National survey of hospital pharmaceutical services — 1978." *American Journal of Hospital Pharmacy* 36: 316–325.

Temin, Peter. 1980. *Taking Your Medicine: Drug Regulation in the United States*. Cambridge, Mass.: Harvard University Press.

Watkins, Roland L. and G. Joseph Norwood. 1978. "Pharmacists drug consultation behavior." *Social Science and Medicine*: 12 (July) 235–239.

Still in the shadow of medicine, all three new health-care providers can be compared according to whether they (1) seek greater autonomy and responsibility; (2) have the likelihood of achieving independent billing even when in supervised practice; and (3) can become part of the profession of medicine as other specialties, such as anesthesiology, radiology, and pathology, or can receive parity status through changing educational requirements as in the case of osteopathy.

Future Directions

Physician Assistants

At the end of the 1980s, it appears that the least volatile of the three new roles is that of physician assistant. A successful innovation from the point of view of its medical sponsors, the role also has been subject to medical specialization. Although limited in both depth and breadth of services, the physician assistant has been used to implement cost containment and manpower distribution policy — slowing down the growth of specialization in medicine by eliminating the need for some house officers in hospitals. This step toward increased specialization for PAs is the most powerful indicator of acceptance of this role that the medical profession can provide. Furthermore, trained PAs are not competitors of existing specialists and, unlike nurse practitioners, they will remain in their present jobs rather than become managers, supervisors, or coordinators. The PAs also have no history of litigious behavior. They cannot be described as participating in a collective mobility project, even though the roles may represent individual social mobility for its performers. As a junior profession, PAs dance to medicine's tune, and remain in its shadow, and they have not developed any organized occupational group seeking to become upwardly mobile.

In the future, I expect that PAs will have a tougher time replacing physicians in primary care. In some ways, PAs are on a collision course with doctors caught up in an oversupply situation. At the same time, HMOs which deliver comprehensive care to subscribers at a prepaid fixed price, find both PAs and NPs attractive providers to hire, since they are less expensive to employ than physicians and can do most of the tasks involved in the delivery of primary care.

The structure of recruitment into medicine and its culture may yet make it possible for the mitigation of competition between PAs and medical doctors. A key factor is the decline in medical school applications and enrollments. With fewer students in medical school, the problem may not be too intense. Primary care is not very appealing to most doctors, both because of the comparatively lower incomes and the repetition of simple problems in the work. Many internists find this work unchallenging. Medical students who choose family practice as their specialty are a very unusual breed in American medical circles. Foreign medical school graduates, may be the major source of competition with PAs because they are happy to practice any kind of medicine and receive adequate remuneration.

In many ways, the current situation of the physician assistant is reminiscent of the beginnings of hospital nursing, with the delegation of tasks regarded by the subordinates as appropriate, instead of whetting their appetites for more responsibility and authority. Surely the tasks they perform are sufficiently important in the delivery of health care to warrant further quests for professionalization.

Nurse Practitioners

Perhaps a more complex situation presents itself when we attempt to predict the future of nurse practitioners (NPs), given their attempt to break out of the limited roles assigned to them by most doctors and their ambivalent relationship with nursing leadership. Nursing appears to be a profession engaging in a collective mobility project of its own, independent of the existence of nurse practitioners. The successful introduction of nurse practitioners came about, not because of the nursing leadership, but in spite of it. Nurse practitioners are now only the most innovative and aggressive wing of nursing, not marginal to the profession as they once were.

The attitudes of nursing leaders are ambivalent toward this new profession. Nurse practitioners can be considered simply stalking horses for nursing leadership. From the perspective of the officers of the ANA and other organizations representing the profession, NPs get to do things that all nurses are capable of doing — only they get to do them first. According to nursing leaders, NPs get recognition for things that nurses have been doing for years, but to date these tasks have not been identified and named as highly skilled, responsible, and autonomous activities. These are some of the rhetorical responses to NPs, but they merely belittle their achievements and fail to recognize their extreme lack of monetary and social rewards for the tasks they accomplish. The pioneer NPs felt limited by the traditional roles in nursing; they wanted to get more deeply into clinical work with patients.

There is a paradox here. The real focus of this quest was not collective mobility but individual growth. Although willing to do comprehensive primary care, NPs did not want to do routine tasks all their working days. The focus on personal growth and autonomy is evidenced by the fact that only half the trained NPs now work in NP roles. The others, have moved into more, not less, responsible positions.

On a personal level, NPs who work in teaching hospitals are particularly well positioned to aspire to higher status and more income. They often spend time training medical students and house officers, who then gain competency and come back to supervise *them*. NPs have told me that they know they are as competent as these doctors, but their mobility is limited; they cannot be appointed directors of medical units because they do not have medical degrees. It is no small wonder that NPs seek to establish independent practices in order to find self-actualization, since so many of the managerial positions in clinical work are closed to them. They have also cut themselves off from management positions in nursing by the presence of their strong clinical orientation. It is obvious that feminist culture is an important factor in nursing and continues to have an impact, particulary among the upwardly mobile.

Motivation for achievement among nurses has an affinity with some important opportunities in health-care delivery. In clinical areas, NPs are well positioned to assume the many counseling and educational tasks that make up a great deal of pediatric practice. The behavioral side of pediatrics is an area where NPs excel, being especially good at counseling young mothers. A renewed concern with the health needs of America's children has emerged, reflecting the neglect of children often observed in this society. A higher proportion of children now live in poverty than any other age group in our society. They make up 40 percent of this sector of the population (Tolchin 1988, E5). At one time, school health services made sure that children's health was not neglected, regardless of parental concern or competency. Now the concern is proactive:

> The key to cost-effective high quality health care for children is child health supervision with its preventive component. However, an inadequate understanding of the health-care needs of children and of the effects of insurance on the financing of their health care has led the health insurance industry to resist coverage of child health supervision. (Austin 1984, 1117)

As the focus shifts to human development and the management of chronic illness, it would seem that nursing in general, and NPs in particular, will move toward performing educational roles. Is this not the direction in which a chronic-disease-oriented profession of medicine ought to go as well? Perhaps the leadership in health care might come from providers who recognize the psychosocial dynamics of health care most acutely. Doctors who initiate home-care programs or develop preventive interventions with the at-risk population are good examples of the behavioral side of medical practice. My colleagues at Albert Einstein College of Medicine — Ruth Stein, Michael Cohen and Henry Ireys — are practitioners with sensitivity to the consequences of families dynamics and their importance to the delivery of effective health care.

In sum, the emerging division of labor in health care – as identified in this kind of conceptualization – is highly receptive to the mobility quest of women. Nurse practitioners, I predict, will achieve greater autonomy only if the delivery of primary care is treated as a serious medical specialty. Working with doctors trained in family medicine, who have learned to work closely with the new health-care practitioners, NPs will be able to have more control over their work. When this happens, the goals of medicine will be articulated more with the larger social purpose of responsibility for the health of all Americans.

Clinical Pharmacy

The larger social purpose of clinical pharmacy is also related to the effectiveness of health-care delivery. As depicted in the rise of clinical pharmacy, a collective mobility project can move in several different directions. Whatever functions are performed – whether technical, clinical or entrepreneurial – pharmacy will still be part of the health-care scene. What is unclear is what social standing pharmacy will have. At the moment, clinical pharmacy is joined in the larger enterprise of licensed dispensing of pharmaceuticals, a profession seen by most observers as secondary to medicine and, for some, as less important than nursing.

The future situation of pharmacy may change, depending on the direction finally taken by the collective mobility project of clinical pharmacy. Several divergent outcomes are possible: (1) an overall upgrading of pharmacy to a clinical profession; (2) the segmentation of clinical pharmacy within the larger profession, with shared authority with physicians limited to hospital and ambulatory-care settings; or (3) an inward-looking profession, concerned with receiving respect. Underlying these possibilities is a concern with social standing, or status. It is useful to consider how to define status, since I am taking a concept based on looking at interaction but showing how it applies directly to more stabilized social relationships. Status can be part of a system of generalized expectations, and therefore the giving or withholding of it is not a matter of individual choice.

Failure to recognize someone's status is insulting to the person, whether of superior or inferior status. Theodore David Kemper (1979), defines status as "a scalar expression of the amount of voluntary compliance an actor or group generally receives or is entitled to from other actors or groups. Status is thus accorded to actors or conferred by actors on other actors."

There is every indication that the field of health care has its own status system. Physicians, for example, are accorded status on both an individual and an organizational level. A physician who receives a hospital appointment will be written about in local newspapers; a nurse who changes jobs will receive no notice. The local junior executive who makes a corporate move will be discussed on the business pages of the community newspaper; the secretary will not. Within the everyday world of health care, an attending physician (one with a hospital appointment) can more easily get to see the director of a hospital on short notice than a nurse, intern, or resident. Furthermore, within the profession of medicine, surgeons are given more respect than doctors who are public health officers.

It has often been said about organizational life that rank deserves respect. Outside the bureaucracy, professional status can be seen as receiving due regard. It is also the case that professional status has its pecuniary rewards. The pharmacist, as well as the physician, can translate status into higher earnings. The pharmacist in a community setting who retails over-the-counter products puts a professional seal of approval on the items sold, whether they are helpful to the consumer or not. The prestige of pharmacy is also exploited in television commercials, as men in white, with the appropriate maturity and somber mien to enhance their appearance, sell dandruff shampoo, balm for hemorrhoids, or "cures" for athlete's foot. While no organizational endorsement is mentioned, suffering customers are relieved to know that the pharmacist stands behind this or that product.

Clinical pharmacists are hardly in a position to turn their status into pecuniary advantage, not because of their rejection of the drug store but because status is based on consensus, a condition that takes time to build. No occupation can confer status on itself. What happens when a profession comes on the scene? When few people recognize the profession's contribution to the common good, it is not easy to turn the status of being among the educated to pecuniary advantage. Too busy and not well enough known to spin off monetary rewards, clinical pharmacists emphasize proving themselves. Concern with image is closely connected with this objective. Larson (1977) hypothesizes that "in the newer professions, the creation, expression and protection of special status tend to be the most central dimensions of the professionalization project" (p. 236). In earlier chapters, I demonstrated the extreme concern shown by the reformers in the field about pharmacy education, ethics and practices, providing evidence in support of Larson's assertion.

Yet pharmacy, is a venerable profession. How does it come about that this ancient profession is still concerned with attaining status? The search for status is not an empty ritual but a campaign to protect the occupation from downgrading. This form of protection operates on both a practical and an ideological level. In practice it can be seen as a response to financial, technical, and organizational changes that threaten pharmacy; reprofessionalization has been advocated within its ranks. This is not an unusual response on the part of professions; when under threat, the prophetic C. Wright Mills (1951) wrote, they "seek to monopolize their positions by closing up their ranks; they seek to do so by law and by stringent rules of education and entrance. Wherever there is a feeling of declining opportunity, occupational groups will seek such closure" (p. 150).

Such an observation may shock readers who idealize professionals. Professionals, by definition, are supposed to be enlightened; when it becomes apparent that a profession is no longer needed, they are supposed to give way to a more rational and efficient system. Like nomads, they are expected to fold their tents and move on. Yet any stable system benefits those who command it. The impact of the fear of loss of status and power often works paradoxically, producing support for the *status quo* rather than a challenge to it. Writing after World War II, at a time of the great transformation of American society, C. Wright Mills focused on the "status panic" of those in the middle class whose positions were being undermined by changes over which they had no control. The emergence of large corporations were restricting the independence of white-collar workers and introducing a reduction in their social status.

Pharmacy is going through a similar process. Reprofession-alization depends on a willingness to take risks in order to gain respect and new responsibilities. Risk taking is not simply doing things differently or expanding one's role; it is making com-parisons — showing what education and ability can do — even when the occupational title would lead others to hold to a very different set of expectations. To break through these old expec-tations, more than successful demonstrations are required; cons-tant comparisons are made between clinical pharmacists and others. Advocates of clinical pharmacy say how they are different from older pharmacists, community pharmacists, nurses, and even doctors. *Different* does mean *better* in the context of these discus-sions. But the statements made are prescriptive, concerning where the profession, according to some, ought to be headed.

What is willed, Friedrich Engels wrote, rarely happens. There is no guarantee that an upgraded profession will follow the remaking of pharmacy. In calling attention to their skills and knowledge, clinical pharmacists seek to be accorded a new status, one commensurate with their functions. They may actually receive this new recognition, not as the new profession of pharmacy or even as a distinctly elite specialty within it, but as a new branch of medicine. An expanded division of labor, recognizing the im-portance of the rational use of drugs, is possible. Medicine has absorbed nonclinical specialties in the past; it has also accorded medical parity, if not equal status, to some alternative providers. A similar outcome is possible for clinical pharmacy. Previous ex-perience suggests that this will mean that pharmacists of the clinical variety will have to have a medical education in addition to pharmacy education.

The New Division of Labor

The relative stabilization of physician assistants in their niches in HMOs and as replacements for house staff, and the turbulence in nursing and ferment in pharmacy, help create a changed and continuously changing status order in health care. The status order itself, as Larson (1977) reminds us, blocks from our vision other realities in an advanced capitalist society.

> As the labor force tends to become totally subsumed under the formal relations of capitalist production, the real and ideological privileges associated with "professionalism" legitimize the class structure by introducing status differentials, status aspirations, and status mobility at practically all levels of the occupational hierarchy. (p. 239)

What Larson means is that the presence of status differences creates the appearance of opportunities for social mobility as opposed to sharp class differences. Thus, the professions, because of their high status, mask the class nature of capitalist society.

This view of things needs a closer look. Status creates its own conflicts. The sources of differentiation are also sources of reevaluations and new understandings within the health-care field, and eventually the sources of institutional change. Some of these day-to-day struggles in the workplace and battles in the courts challenge the professional dominance of medicine. Insofar as this changing division of labor involves a transfer of decision making as well as responsibilities, then social change is occurring. Without power over resources, including how tasks are to be distributed in a division of labor, there can be no serious change in the division of labor in health care. Access to the use of important rights, such as hospital admissions and prescribing, means that physician extenders and clinical pharmacists can carry out their responsibilities. I would have to agree with Alford (1972) that

> . . . medicine seems to be a classic case of the socialization of production but the private appropriation of the "surplus" by a vested interest group—the doctors—who maintain control through their professional associations of the supply of physicians, the distribution of services, the cost of services and the rules governing hospitals. (p. 142)

The continued rise in expenditures for health care in the United States, now reaching 12 percent of the GNP (Freudenheim, 1988), makes these institutional arrangements hopelessly old-fashioned and expensive from the point of view of American capitalists, who wish to socialize the means of medical and health production for their own ends. When it comes to considering how to become more competitive with other advanced industrial nations in the world , cost containment means reducing fringe benefits. And the charges for medical benefits are out of control.

There appear to be struggles within struggles here. On another level, the creation of new health-care practitioners points to new developments and refinements in the struggles between people without power, resulting from structured accumulated disadvantage. Elliot Krause noted (1977) that "the social class distinctions of the wider society are reproduced in the way different social groups — by sex, race and social class — are tracked into the division of labor in health work" (p. 42).

Under what conditions do professional developments represent a change in class position and status? Is status enhancement without change in real income and other bases of power merely the appearance of change? Does a decline in status, or the threat of a decline, make more apparent the class nature of capitalist society, by stripping away its masks? And is the reverse true: Can an occupational upgrade make actors in society feel that society is not fixed and frozen in class relationships?

I cannot answer these questions here. Yet, despite the limits to this study, I will not dismiss all the changes in the division of labor in health care as merely superstructural and not of deeper structural significance. Status distinctions sometimes represent more significant work redesign efforts. Along this line of inquiry, I have to consider the importance of even partial autonomy as a form of empowerment. Many of the new health-care practitioners believe that their work has purpose. And this helps answer one of the compelling modern questions concerning whether work under increasing specialization and technologic development will provide the satisfactions it once did.

The new health-care practitioners also make possible — at a reasonable cost — effective primary care, delivered in a personalized fashion. Americans want a personalized relationship with health-care providers and value those that they currently have. Despite all the cynicism about health-care providers, especially the profession of medicine, Americans *trust* their doctors. They do not trust powerful and distant institutions.

Perhaps this is a carryover from the Progressive era when the first reforms of medicine took place.

The quality of life today is definitely enhanced when we can say we have a regular source of care. Health care can be life giving and life enhancing; in a complementary way, professional workers grow as the result of this problem solving and support for people in need. We all need to be reminded, as the nineteenth-century physician Virchow advocated, that medicine is a social and not a natural science.

Finally, it is significant that this study is not just a look at the struggles of the new health care practitioners and clinical pharmacists but of the self-generating capacity for change found in the behavior and ideas of the performers of these roles. The quest for autonomy, even as a response to structural changes that are a threat to traditional practices, is in itself, a dynamic in the health care field. The division of labor will continue to change, reflecting tensions between circumstances and human responses to them. The outcomes will continue to shape and challenge that division of labor.

References

Alford, R.1972. "The political economy of health care: Dynamics without change." *Politics and Society* (Winter): 1–38.

Austin, G. 1984. "Sounding board: Child health-care financing and competition." *New England Journal of Medicine* 75: 1117–1120.

Freudenheim, Milton. 1988. "U.S. health care spending continues sharp rise." *New York Times* (November 19): 1, 50.

Kemper, Theodore D. 1979. "Why are the streets so dirty?" *Social Forces* 58: 422–442.

Krause, Elliott. 1977. *Power and Illness: The Political Sociology of Health and Medical Care*. New York: Elsevier.

Larson, Margali Safatti. 1977. *The Rise of Professionalism*. Berkeley: University of California Press.

Mills, C. Wright. 1951. *White Collar*. New York: Oxford University Press.

Tolchin, Martin. 1988. "Generational issues: What's fair to the young and the taxed?" *New York Times* (November 27): E5.

Name Index

Adamcik, B., 47, 53, 148, 154
Aiken, Linda, 100
Alford, Robert, 106, 116
Altman, Lawrence, 149, 150, 164, 166
Anderson, P.O., 131, 135
American Association of Colleges of Pharmacy, 141
American Druggist, 115
American Journal of Hospital Pharmacy (AJHP), 121, 122, 124
American Medical Association (AMA), 59, 73
American Society of Hospital Pharmacists (ASHP) Board, 114, 116, 127
Angorn, R.A., 107, 116
Applied Management Sciences, 111, 116
Ashikaga, T., 67, 75
Austin, G., 159, 166

Barber, Elinor, 14, 15
Barnhart, Rick, 152, 153, 154
Barofsky, I., 137, 138
Barton, Clara, 34
Batey, M.V., 85, 99
Baumgartner, R.P., Jr., 130, 131, 135
Becker, Howard, 63, 73
Becker, M.H., 120, 136
Beckhard, R., 35, 53
Begun, J.W., 44, 54
Bevins, G.M., 104, 116
Birenbaum, Arnold, 63, 73, 103, 115, 116, 144, 145, 154
Bliss, A.A., 56, 73

Bologh, Roslyn, 144, 145, 154
Boor, M., 130, 137
Brands, A.J., 129, 136
Braverman, Harry, 50, 54
Breslau, N., 93, 99
Broadhead, Robert S., 44, 54, 118, 136
Brodie, D.C., 110, 116
Brouwer, H., 120, 137
Brown, M.S., 82, 99
Burkett, G.L., 80, 99
Bush, P.J., 47, 54

Cable, G., 130, 138
Cambridge Research Institute (CRI), 38, 40, 54, 56, 58, 73
Campagna,K.D., 139
Carter, W.B., 120, 136
Catizone, C., 136
Cawley, J.F., 60, 73
Charney, E., 92, 99
Cheyovich, T.K., 62, 74, 82, 100
Choi, M.W., 81, 99
Christansen, D.B., 47, 54
Cihlar, C., 40, 54
Claiborn, S.A., 79, 99
Clore, E.R., 62, 74
Cohen, Michael, 159
Coleman, J.H., 3rd, 132, 136
Collins, Wilkie, 17, 31
Conrad, Peter, 155
Contemporary Pharmacy Practice, 115
Corley, J.B., 82, 100
Covington, R.R., 129, 136
Creighton, Helen, 96, 99
Crouch, V., 68, 74
Cruikshank, B.M., 67, 73
Curtiss, F.R., 144, 154

167

Davies, L.R., 72, 74
daVinci, Leonardo, 16
Davins, D., 130, 137
Day, L.R., 61, 74
Denzin, Norman K., 3, 15, 47, 54
Dichter Institute, 105, 116
Dickson, W. Michael, 152, 154
DeMarco, C.T., 123, 136
deWolf, P.L., 69, 74, 96, 101
Duncan, B., 69, 73, 91, 101
Durkheim, Emile, 5

Ehrenreich, Barbara, 28, 31
Ehrenreich, John, 28, 31
Engels, Friedrich, 163
Enggist, R.E., 92, 99
Evans, R.L., 132, 136

Facchinetti, N.J., 44, 54, 118, 137,
    152, 154
Feldman, R.D., 44, 54
Fink, J.L. III, 123, 136
Fisk, P.A., 132, 138
Fletcher C., 120, 136
Flexner, Abraham, 28
Ford, L.C., 61, 74
Forrest, T.P., 123, 138
Foster, T.S., 110, 117
Fowler, E.H., 77, 99
Fox, J.G., 93, 94, 99
Francke, Donald E., 3, 15, 109,
    111, 116, 125, 126, 136
Fraser, C.H., 91, 101
Freeborn, D.K., 80, 100
Freidson, Eliot, 19, 21, 22, 24, 31,
    63, 65, 66, 73, 103, 108, 116
Freud, Sigmund, 70
Freudenheim, Milton, 164, 166

Gagnon, John Paul, 48
Gay, Peter, 70, 73
Gallina, J.N., 108, 116
Geer, B., 63, 73
Gieryn, T.F., 104, 105, 116, 119,
    136
Gillings, D.B., 80, 100
Girard, D.E., 120, 137
Glascock, J.C., 67, 73

Glaser, M., 51, 54
Glazer, W., 39, 54
Goddard, James L., 151, 155
Goffman, Erving, 11, 15
Golden, A.S., 60, 74
Goldstein, E., 129, 136
Goleman, D., 70, 73
Goyan, Jere E., 45, 46
Graduate Medical Education
    National Advisory Commit-
    tee, 56, 68, 74, 79, 99
Graham, A.W., 130, 138
Grauer, D.W., 121, 136
Greenberg, S., 82, 99
Greifinger, Robert, 28, 31
Greiner, G.E., 127, 136

Haigh, V.H., 136
Halster, J., 137
Hammel, R.J., 144, 154, 155
Hanlon, C.R., 83, 99
Hartoum, H.T., 120, 136
Hatcher, M.E., 92, 99
Hauser, L.D., 131, 135
Hayden, M.L., 62, 74
Haynes, R.B., 120, 136
Health Services Research Center,
    92, 99
Heinen, J.S., 144, 154, 155
Heller, W.M., 125, 136
Henderson, H.R., 130, 137
Hogan, K.A., 93, 99
Hogan, R.A.,93, 99
Holbrook, T.L., 94, 101
Holcomb, B., 48, 54
Holland, J.M., 85, 99
Hughes, Everett C., 12, 15
Hutchinson, R.A., 47, 55, 136

Iacocca, Lee, 29
Institute of Medicine, 41, 54
Inui, T.S., 136
Ireys, Henry, 159
Ivey, M.F., 110, 116, 130, 132,
    136, 137

James, J., 74
Jaspars, J., 120, 137

Jeffrey, L.P., 108, 117, 125, 137
Jinks, M., 130, 137
Johnson, E.A., 144, 154, 155
Johnson, R.E, 80, 100, 131, 137
Johnson, Terrance, 22, 31

Kane, R.L., 82, 100
Keefer, C.S., 122, 137
Kemper, Theodore D., 161, 166
Kern, Rochelle, 155
Kidder, S.W., 131, 137
Kirk, R.F., 136
Kissner, E.A., 131, 137
Kitzman, H., 92, 99
Klegon, D., 43, 54
Kolbert, E., 95, 100
Kormel, B., 47, 54
Kotelchuch, David, 154
Knapp, D.A., 48, 54
Knapp, D.E., 48, 49, 54
Knox, G.K., 60, 74
Krause, Elliott, 165, 166
Kronus, C., 44, 47, 54, 141, 155
Kukull, W.A., 136
Kviz, F.J., 93, 100

Lairson, P., 69, 74
Lakin, J.A., 67, 73
Lamb, G.S., 82, 100
Lamy, P.O., 3, 15, 47, 54
Land, M.J., 85, 100, 131, 135
LaPlante, L.J., 85, 100
Larkin, Gerald, 26, 31
Larson, Margalie Safatti, 17, 31,
        52, 54, 103, 104, 117, 118,
        137, 142, 148, 155, 162,
        163, 166
Lawrence, R.S., 80, 100
Ledwoch, W., 130, 138
Lee, Philip R., 131, 137
Leeds,N.H., 139, 145
Lesieur, Henry, 144, 145, 154
Levine, D.M., 82, 100
Lewin, K., 122, 138
Lewis, C.E., 62, 74, 82, 100
Light, D.W., 41, 54, 79, 100
Linn, L.S., 93, 100
Lipton, Helene L., 131, 137

Little, M., 80, 81, 100
Lorber, Judith, 15
Love, D.W., 47, 54
Lukacs, J.L., 68, 74
Lyons, R.C., 45, 46, 54

Manber, M.M., 72, 74
Marston, M.V., 120, 137
Marx, Karl, 5, 6, 32, 142, 155
McAtee, P.A., 82, 101
McCarthy, A.M., 67, 73
McCormack, T.H., 122, 138
McDonald, J., 136
McKeown, Thomas, 27, 31
McKenny, J.M., 130, 137
McKinley, J.D. Jr, 130, 138
McLeod, D.C., 138
McMath, J.C., 120, 137
Mechanic, David, 47, 49, 55, 90,
        100
Mehl, B., 131, 137
Meinhold, J.M., 47, 55
Merton, Robert K., 14, 15, 49, 55
Miller, D.E., 110, 117
Millis, J., 111, 117
Mills, C. Wright, 162, 166
Misener, T.R., 93, 100
Miyagawa, C.I., 128, 137
Mueller, W., 130, 136

Napodano, R.J., 82, 100
Nardone, D.A., 120, 137
National Associations of Boards of
        Pharmacy, 48, 50, 55
National Center for Health
        Statistics, 36, 55
Nelson, A.A., 47, 55
Neuhauser, Duncan, 56, 74
Nightingale, Florence, 34
Noordenbus, A., 74
Norwood, G. Joseph, 144, 155
Novack, A.H., 93, 99

O'Bannon, F.V., 85, 100
Ott, J.E., 60, 74

Parsons, Talcott, 18, 21, 31
Pathak, D.S., 139

Pearson, Linda, J., 96, 100
Pender, A.R., 94, 100
Pender, N.J., 94, 100
Pendleton, D.A., 120, 137
Perrow, Charles, 152, 155
Pfeiffer, F.G., 129, 136
Pharmaceutical Director, 114
Pierce, M., 82, 100
Platt, F.W., 120, 137
Poulantzas, Nicolas, 29, 31
Provost, G.P., 45, 50, 55, 106,
        108, 113, 114, 117, 121,
        124, 125, 126, 127, 138,
        146, 155
Puckett, F.J., 115, 117
Purohit, A., 136

Quattlebaum, T.G., 82, 100

Raehl, C.L., 110, 117
Raney, M.R., 148, 155
Rapson, M.F., 67, 74
Rawlings, J.L., 132, 138
Ray, Max, 143, 155
Record, J., 74
Reeve, Henry, 15
Reinders, T.P., 130, 138
Reiser D.E., 120, 138
Reuler, J.B., 120, 137
Richards, R.W., 138
Riella, M. , 130, 136
Ritchey, F.J.,148, 155
Rivera, J.O., 128, 137
Robbins, J., 115, 117
Robertson, W.J., 84, 100
Rodeghero, J.A., 92, 100
Rosenberg, Charles, 32, 33, 55
Rosenbluth, S.A., 132, 135
Rueschemeyer, D., 21, 31
Ruggiero, J.S., 113, 117
Rush, D.R., 130, 138

Sackett, D.L., 120, 136
Sadler, A.M., 56, 74
Sadler, B.L., 56, 74
Sager, Alan, 30, 31
Saward, E.W., 59, 74
Scheffler, R.M., 80, 100

Schilling, L.S., 94, 101
Schiff, D.W., 91, 101
Schneider, P., 130, 138
Schroder, A.D., 120, 138
Schrey, A., 130, 138
Schwartz, H.D., 69, 74, 96, 101
Schwartz, M.A., 3, 15, 120, 138
Scribner, B., 130, 136
Shamansky, S.L., 94, 101
Sharpe, T.R., 120, 138
Shaw, George Bernard, 18
Sidel, Victor, 28, 31
Silver, H.K., 60, 61, 74, 91, 101
Silver, H.S., 82, 101
Silver, George, 23, 31, 40, 55, 57,
        74
Skipper, J.K., 69, 74, 96, 101
Slining, J.M., 130, 137
Smith, C.W., 92, 101
Smith, D.W., 94, 101
Smith, M.D., 49, 55, 110, 117
Snoke, Albert W., 70, 73
Spitzer, W.O., 85, 96, 101
Spunt, A.L., 139
Starkweather, D.B., 35, 55
Stamm, K., 110, 117
Starr, Paul, 9, 10, 12, 13, 15, 25,
        31, 118, 138
Stead, Eugene A., 59
Stearly, S., 68, 74
Steeves, R.F., 123, 138
Stein, Ruth, 61, 159
Stephens, S.P., 130, 138
Steton, D., 57, 74
Stolar, M.H., 127, 138, 143, 155
Storms, D.M., 93, 94, 99
Sullivan, J.A., 85, 101
Sullivan, R., 70, 74

Taffet, S., 70, 74
Talley, C.R., 109, 110, 117, 128,
        138
Taryle, D.A., 131, 135
Taylor, D.W., 120, 136
Temin, Peter, 149, 153, 155
Thompson, E.P., 45, 55
Tocqueville, Alexis de, 6, 15
Tolchin, Martin, 159, 166

Tremblay, J., 110, 117
Truman, Harry S., 13
Tso, Y., 110, 116
Tuchier, R.J., 131, 137
Tucker, Robert, 155

Ure, Andrew, 27, 31
U.S. Congressional Budget Office,
    93, 101
U.S. Department of Health and
    Human Services, 72, 73, 74
U.S. Office of Technology Assess-
    ment, 61, 75, 79, 81, 85, 86,
    89, 101

Vacek, P., 67, 75
Vinson, N., 93,100
Vox Paed, 79, 83, 101

Wagner, J., 129, 138
Walker, P.W., 136
Walters, H.L., 91, 101
Walton, W., 79, 99
Watkins, Roland L., 144, 155
Watanabe, A.S., 110, 117
Weber, Max, 1, 5, 22
Webster-Stratton, C., 67, 73
Weiland, Anne P., 83, 101
West, D.P., 139
Whitney, H.A.K., Jr., 125, 138
Wilson, Florence, 59, 75
Witte, K.W., 132, 139
Worcester, Alfred, 39

Zehr, S.C., 104, 116
Zellmer, William A., 2, 15, 51, 55,
    106, 107, 111, 113, 117,
    127, 139

Subject Index

Bureaucracy:
  complexity of tasks, 35;
  health care, 34;
  hospital size, 35

Clinical pharmacy:
  as a movement, 3;
  boundary work, 104–105,
    118–139;
  collective mobility project,
    104–121;
  comparison to physician
    associates, 53;
  creating markets for services,
    121–134;
  cultural authority of, 3, 13,
    118–139;
  definition, 2;
  efforts to create a consistent
    image, 103–116;
  future directions, 160–163;
  increasing professionalism in
    associations, 113–114;
  opportunities to practice,
    140–149;
  physician response, 148;
  preventing adverse drug affects,
    24

Diagnostic Related Groups
  (DRGs), 58

Experts:
  functions, 14, 17;
  uncertainty, 23;

Health care system:
  capital intensive field, 41;
  cost containment efforts, 42;

expansion of services, 76;
labor intensive field, 41;
new division of labor, 163–166;
proliferation of employment,
  58;
specialties, 58;
task shifting, 42;
technology, 58
Health Maintenance Organizations
  (HMOs), 41:
  prepaid plans, 58;
  prospective payment systems,
    42
Hospitals:
  as complex organizations (see
    bureaucracies) 32, 35;
  and the marketplace, 33;
  technological advances, 34;
  as physicians' workshops, 35;
  team approach to care, 35;
  task delegation, 59;

Institution:
  definition, 11;

Medicine:
  autonomy, 26;
  control, 26;
  corporate rationalizers, 31, 40,
    56;
  creation of physician extender
    roles, 78;
  dependent professions, 30;
  high technology, 23;
  impact on general labor supply,
    27;
  material foundation of cultural
    authority, 149–154;

nested professions,30;
primary care shortages, 37–38;
social integration functions, 28;
social reproduction, 27, 29;
sovereign profession, 30;
specialization, 4, 23;
task delegation, 57
Middle-level health-care practitioners (see physician extenders, nurse practitioners,
and physician assistants),
38–39

Nested professions, 30
Nurse Practitioners:
autonomy 66–67;
boundary encroachment, 68,
70;
community practice, 95–97;
creditability, 84;
direct payment to, 97;
education and training, 60–61,
67;
evaluation of performance, 69,
85–90;
future directions, 157–160;
independent judgment, 65, 67;
information dispensing, 63;
institutional licensing, 78;
legal restrictions on practice,
68, 72, 96;
new tasks, 67;
patient satisfaction, 90–95;
pediatric practice, 83;
physician approval, 79–82;
professional identity formation,
62;
recruitment, 61–62;
sense of responsibility, 4, 63;
uncertainty, 67–68

Pharmacy:
clinical roles (see Clinical
pharmacy);
crisis in pharmacy, 43–45, 47;
elites in pharmacy, 45;
fear of displacement, 45, 105;
lack of unity, 46;

reforms in education, 143–148;
reprofessionalization, 114–116;
structural changes, 47–52
Physician assistants:
boundary encroachment, 72;
education and training, 40, 59;
evaluation of performance, 85;
future directions, 156–157;
independent judgment, 77;
institutional licensing, 78;
negotiated autonomy, 72;
patient satisfaction, 91–95;
physician acceptance, 40,
79–82;
practice location, 41;
recruitment, 40;
sense of responsibility, 4;
utilization, 82–84;
utilization restrictions, AMA,
71
Physician associates (see nurse
practitioners and physician
assistants), 40:
task shifting, 42;
Physician Clinical Associates,
(PCA), 83
Physician extenders, 2:
acceptance by doctors, 77;
autonomy, 24;
Child Health Associates, 60;
cognitive credibility, 69, 84;
future directions, 156–160;
negotiated autonomy, 71;
patient approval, 77;
physician shortage, 36;
relationship to physicians, 77,
79;
reducing hospital bed use, 38;
Prevention of disease:
nutrition, 27;
public health, 28
Professions:
coordinating and control
functions, 12;
collective mobility projects, 52;
corporate groups, 18;
credentials, 24;
division of labor, 26;

government support, 21–22;
group mobility, 22;
labor market shelters, 24;
legitimation, 8, 12, 18, 19, 20;
medical domination and
    control, 11, 19, 21;
modern society, 17, 18;
normative force, 16–20, 28;
origins and conditions for
    emergence, 5;
Progressive Era, 29;
reprofessionalization, 52;
self-regulation, 19, 23;

sovereign professions, 25
Professional characteristics:
    information dispensing, 63;
    independent judgment, 5, 23,
        65;
    sense of responsibility, 63

Self-insurance:
    price negotiation, 41

Sociology of Occupations and
        Professions:
    methodological problems, 7–10

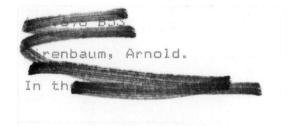